*Fibroid
Tumors &
Endometriosis*

✦ ✦ ✦

Fibroid Tumors & Endometriosis

♦ ♦ ♦

Susan M. Lark, M.D.

Westchester Publishing Company
Los Altos, California

Cover & Text Design: Brad Greene
Photographs: Ronald May
Illustrations: Shelly Reeves Smith
Printing & Binding: Arcata Graphics Company

International Standard Book Number: 0-917010-54-X
Library of Congress Catalog Card Number: 93-60452

Westchester Publishing Company
342 State Street, Suite 6
Los Altos, CA 94022
415-941-5784

To my wonderful husband Jim and
my darling daughter Rebecca
To the health and well-being of all women

✦ ✦ ✦

Contents

Introduction

A Self-Help Approach
to Fibroids & Endometriosis

*F*ibroids and endometriosis are diseases that affect many women during their prime reproductive years, most often from their twenties through their forties. These are the years when women are starting and developing their careers and families—a time of new and exciting life experiences. Energy and a zest for life are often at their peak. These women work at energy levels they may never achieve again; though many will remain active into their older years, they will tend to live more sensibly and at a more moderate pace.

Yet, for the millions of younger women who suffer from symptoms caused by fibroids or endometriosis, the quality of life often declines significantly. These women have recurrent painful and unpleasant symptoms that jeopardize their ability to work, care for children, enjoy personal relationships, and even engage in sexual intercourse during a period of several days to several weeks each month. Fibroids and endometriosis are common causes of infertility and affect the ability of some women to bear children.

Although the actual disease processes are quite different— fibroids are benign tumors in the uterus, while endometriosis is a condition that causes inflammation and scarring in the pelvis—they are often triggered by the same mechanisms. Hormonal imbalances, stress, and nutritional factors play major roles in both problems. Why some women develop one disease rather than the other or why other women develop both diseases at the same time is not known. Symptoms of the two diseases are fairly similar. As a result, they are often treated by the same types of drugs and surgical procedures, although the overlap is certainly not total.

Women with severe fibroids or endometriosis have historically been treated with many different drug and hormonal therapies in an attempt to control the symptoms. These women faced a high risk of eventually having a hysterectomy. Luckily, women today can often avoid this grim scenario. A healthy lifestyle can play a beneficial role in relieving and preventing the symptoms of fibroids and endometriosis. New medical therapies that have become available during the past 15 years are more effective than those used in the past. I discuss both the self-care and medical therapies for fibroids and endometriosis in great detail in this book. All women with symptoms caused by these two diseases can look forward to relief by following a more modern therapeutic approach that is grounded strongly in self-help techniques and good medical care.

Learning to Help My Patients

Over the past 20 years, I have worked with many patients who suffered from fibroids and endometriosis. Many of my patients have benefited from a self-care approach to their problems. While medication and even surgery may be necessary to treat women with more advanced disease, the importance of practicing beneficial lifestyle habits cannot be underestimated for symptom relief and prevention. I have spent years researching the use of diet, nutrition, and many other techniques as part of a complete approach to treating these problems. I have learned specific acupressure points, yoga stretches, exercise routines, and various approaches to stress management in order to give my patients many different self-care options. My goal with patients has always been to provide the information, education, and resources to help them relieve their symptoms through becoming healthier women and then maintaining this state through healthy lifestyle practices. I have been delighted with the positive feedback that my patients give me. They are always pleased and relieved to find that self-help treatments are so beneficial and effective.

How to Use This Book

I feel strongly that any woman interested in self-care should have access to this information. Because there are many women whom I will never see as patients in my medical practice, I wrote this book to share with them the self-care techniques that I have found, through many years of medical practice, to be most useful. I hope you will find this information as useful as my patients have. I also practice these techniques. Preventive health care has had tremendous benefits for me; I am healthier and more productive now than I was ten years ago. I plan to feel better and to be even healthier ten years from now. I am continuously expanding my own knowledge about self-help and researching new health-care techniques for treating fibroids and endometriosis.

The fibroid and endometriosis self-help program provides important information for all women suffering from these problems. I have devised the program so that each woman reading this book can select from a wide variety of self-help treatment options. A treatment plan that utilizes only one method and purports to be the only treatment for these two problems will probably work for only a small percentage of women. In my medical practice, I have better results when I individualize each patient's treatment program. By overlapping treatments from various disciplines, most women find a combination that works for them. You will be able to find a combination that works for you, too.

This program is set up to enable you to develop your own treatment plan. All the methods you need are contained in this book. There is information on diet and nutrition, as well as vitamins, minerals, herbs, and essential fatty acids found to be effective for fibroid and endometriosis symptom relief. Nutritional supplementation is an important part of an optimal health program for women facing these health-care problems. Stress reduction techniques, physical exercise, acupressure massage, deep breathing exercises, and yoga positions that are specifically helpful for fibroids and endometriosis are also included. Chapters on drug therapies and surgical procedures for fibroids and endometriosis explain the most effective medical treatments, too.

Read through the entire book first to familiarize yourself with the material. The Fibroid and Endometriosis Workbook (Chapter 3) will help you evaluate your symptoms, your risk factors, and the lifestyle habits that can affect your health. Then turn to the therapy chapters and read through the rest of the book. Try all the therapies that pertain to your symptoms; some will probably make you feel better than others. Establish a regimen that works for you and follow it every day.

This fibroid and endometriosis self-help program is practical and easy to follow. You can use it by itself or in conjunction with a medical program. While working with a physician is necessary to establish a definitive diagnosis of these two problems, and medical therapy may still be necessary for women with moderate to severe symptoms, the importance of a good self-help program cannot be underestimated. For many women, this book can help speed up the diagnostic process. My self-help techniques can play a major role in reducing the severity of your symptoms and preventing recurrences of the disease process. The feeling of wellness that can be yours with a self-help program will radiate out and touch your whole life. You will have more time and energy to enjoy your work, family, and other pleasures in life. Most of my patients tell me that their lives have been positively transformed by these beneficial self-help techniques.

Identifying
the Problem

✦ ✦ ✦

1

What Are Fibroids?

$\mathcal{F}$ibroids are one of the most common female health problems affecting women during their reproductive years. They occur primarily in women in their twenties through their late forties. Their incidence can occasionally extend through menopause, affecting women in their fifties and beyond. Fibroid tumors of the uterus are found in at least 40 percent of American women who reach menopause. Over time, tens of millions of women develop these growths.

Not all fibroids require medical intervention. In fact, many women with fibroids go through years of annual pelvic exams in which the physician simply notes the fibroids on the chart, for they are causing no problems whatsoever. However, approximately 50 percent of women with fibroids develop symptoms severe enough to have a major impact on quality of life. In my practice, fibroids are a very common finding that often coexists with other gynecological complaints such as PMS, menstrual cramps, ovarian cysts, endometriosis, and heavy menstrual flow.

The word *fibroid* is actually a misnomer, because it implies that these tumors arise from fibrous tissue. The correct medical term used by gynecologists for these growths is *leiomyoma* or *myoma*, since these tumors arise from the smooth muscle layer of the uterus (also called the myometrium). This muscle layer lies under the inner lining of the uterus, or endometrium, which bleeds each month during a woman's menstrual period. Since most women are not familiar with the more technical term *leiomyoma*, I will continue to use the term *fibroid* throughout this book.

Fibroids are benign growths that can actually arise in muscle tissue anywhere in the body but are found most commonly in the uterus. Unlike cancer, they do not invade surrounding tissue or distant organs, nor will untreated fibroids kill the affected person. In fact, less than one-half of 1 percent of fibroids ever become cancerous; this usually occurs in postmenopausal women. Instead, these benign muscular tumors tend to remain within the confines of the uterine tissue. However, as they grow larger, they can extend their range and put pressure on neighboring organs and tissues. As the tumor grows, the surrounding tissue is condensed and compressed, forming a type of capsule around the tumor.

Fibroids can vary in number and size. Often multiple fibroids arise over time. Physicians performing surgery on fibroids have found as many as several hundred tumors on a single woman. Fibroids range in size from tiny pinpoint areas of tissue to rare cases of tumors weighing up to 25 pounds or more.

Significant growth of the fibroids usually causes the entire uterus to enlarge. Often a gynecologist feels a firm, irregularly enlarged uterus with smoothly rounded protrusions arising from the uterine wall. Gynecologists tend to describe fibroids in terms of the uterine enlargement caused by pregnancy. A woman with fibroids may be described by her physician as having a "12- to 14-week-size uterus" or even a "20- to 24-week-size uterus," which approximates a 6-month pregnancy in a woman with very large tumors. Interestingly, not all large fibroids cause symptoms. If the fibroids grow in a way that does not cause pressure on neighboring organs, a woman can live with large fibroids for many years without needing medical care.

Most fibroids (95 percent) occur in the body of the uterus; the remaining 5 percent arise from the cervix. Fibroids can arise in different locations within the uterus. *Submucosal* fibroids grow on the inside of the uterus and extend into the uterine cavity from the lining of the uterus, or endometrium. *Intramural* fibroids grow within the uterine wall; *subserosal* fibroids grow on the outside of the uterus, in the lining between the uterus and the pelvic cavity. Some fibroids can grow large enough to extend their boundaries from the uterus into the pelvic ligaments. Each may even develop a long, narrow stalk as it extends into the pelvic cavity. Occasionally fibroids grow large enough to press on the bowel or bladder, or through the cervix, where they can be mistaken for cervical polyps during a gynecological examination. Rarely, they attach to the intestinal wall and become parasitic on the tissue of the bowel lining. Thus, fibroids can grow in a variety of locations from the uterine muscle and can impinge on different pelvic organs depending on their pattern of growth.

Risk Factors That Increase the Likelihood of Fibroids

Fibroids are much more sensitive to estrogen stimulation than is normal muscle tissue. If the tendency toward fibroid tumors exists, stimulation by estrogen can cause these tumors to grow. They can grow rapidly and become very large when estrogen levels are high, such as during pregnancy, or when exposed to birth control pills containing high doses of estrogen. Normally, fibroids shrink and even disappear during menopause when the estrogen levels produced by the body decline greatly. However, the use of estrogen replacement therapy can reactivate and stimulate the growth of fibroids in some postmenopausal women, occasionally leading to severe complications such as heavy menstrual bleeding. Even excessive body weight can increase fibroid growth, because women who are overweight tend to secrete high levels of estrogen.

Fibroids also coexist in women who show other signs of elevated estrogen, such as anovulatory cycles—menstrual cycles in which only estrogen is secreted without progesterone. These cycles are often seen in women under severe emotional and physical stress, during the transition into menopause, or with endometrial hyperplasia (an overgrowth of the uterine lining that occurs when estrogen levels are high). These conditions are associated with an increased risk of uterine cancer. Women with uterine fibroids are also at an increased risk of developing uterine cancer.

Even poor nutritional habits can elevate estrogen levels by inhibiting the body's ability to break down and excrete excess estrogen. The liver has a dual role in digestion—processing the foods that we take in through our daily meals and regulating hormonal levels by deactivating hormones. A high-stress diet—one that is too rich in saturated fats from meats and dairy products, alcohol, sugar, or other difficult-to-handle foods—may overwork the liver, leaving it unable to break down the hormones efficiently. This leads to the elevated levels of estrogen that can trigger fibroids.

Though estrogen is secreted by the ovaries in a form called estradiol, the liver metabolizes estrogen so it can be eliminated from the body effectively, first by converting estradiol to an intermediary form called estrone, and finally to estriol. The liver's ability to efficiently convert estradiol to estriol is important because estriol is the safest and least chemically active form of estrogen. In contrast, estrone and estradiol are very active stimulants of breast and uterine tissue and may worsen estrogen-dependent problems like PMS, fibrocystic breast disease, fibroids, endometriosis, and even breast cancer. Besides metabolizing estrogen to safer forms, the liver helps to keep the levels of estrogen circulating in the blood from getting too high. Thus, healthy liver function is necessary for estrogen metabolism.

The liver is also dependent on an adequate supply of vitamin B to carry out its tasks. If B vitamins are lacking in the diet, the liver does not have the raw materials it needs to perform its metabolic tasks and regulate estrogen levels. (I discuss both diet and nutritional supplementation as treatment for fibroids in Chapters 4, 5, and 6; see those chapters for more detailed information.)

An inherited tendency toward the development of fibroids

seems to exist. Women of African or Asian descent have a two- to fivefold greater risk of developing fibroids than do Caucasian women. The tendency to develop fibroid tumors often runs in families. Many patients tell me that their mothers or sisters have fibroids, too; this is a relatively common story when a physician takes a medical history. Fibroids also seem to be more prevalent in women who haven't had children. Conversely, the more children you have, the less likely you are to develop fibroids.

In summary, though risk factors such as racial and family background cannot be changed, fibroids can be greatly influenced by the hormones we use, the foods we eat, and personal stress. Healthy lifestyle habits can reduce your exposure to such factors. I discuss this subject in great detail in the self-help chapters of this book.

Symptoms of Fibroids

Though many women never have symptoms from fibroids, 50 percent of the women with fibroids require medical help. Depending on size and location, fibroids can cause a variety of symptoms; the most common include bleeding, pain, and infertility. I discuss each of these symptoms in depth in this section. Check with your physician if you have these symptoms and suspect that fibroids could be the cause.

Bleeding. Approximately one-third of women with fibroids suffer from abnormal uterine bleeding. Many women develop heavier menstrual flow that often lasts more days than normal. Some women develop irregular bleeding between periods. In my practice, I have seen women with fibroids develop such heavy bleeding that they actually become anemic. If not treated rapidly, heavy bleeding can cause significant health problems such as weakness, tiredness, and shortness of breath on exertion. If the bleeding continues unchecked, a woman can end up requiring hospitalization and a surgical procedure to stop the problem. Check with your physician if you notice changes in your bleeding pattern. Any significant changes in menstrual flow must be evaluated, since the cause could be rapidly growing fibroids or another serious medical problem.

The most common cause of abnormal bleeding is submucosal fibroids. Submucosal fibroids grow right into the uterine cavity and affect the lining of the uterus, or endometrium. Intramural fibroids, which grow into the wall of the uterus, can worsen bleeding also. There are several reasons why fibroids cause this heavy bleeding pattern. The growth of fibroids may expand the area of the cavity by 10 to 15 times, thus providing a greater surface area to bleed each month. They can also push against the blood vessels in the uterus and disrupt the normal blood flow; this pattern occurs with intramural fibroids. It may be that the presence of an intramural fibroid restricts uterine contractions and interferes with the constriction of the endometrial blood vessels, allowing excessive bleeding.

The high levels of estrogen that stimulate the growth of fibroids can also disrupt normal functioning of the uterine lining. Usually the normal balance between estrogen and progesterone regulates the amount of menstrual blood loss. When estrogen levels are elevated, blood loss from the endometrium increases, adding to the excessive flow already caused by the fibroids.

Pain. Many women with fibroids experience symptoms of pressure and pain, sometimes feeling a sense of progressive pelvic fullness or a dragging sensation. This is most commonly due to slowly enlarging intramural or subserosal fibroids. Such fibroids may be easy to feel during a pelvic or abdominal exam. In fact, my patients with very large fibroids are often astonished at the ease with which they can feel their own fibroids through the abdominal wall.

Fibroids that grow to the point of creating pressure on other pelvic structures may affect both bladder and bowel function. When pressing against the bladder, a fibroid tumor can cause a reduction in bladder capacity, resulting in frequent urination and urgency. Occasionally, pressure on a ureter (the tube that brings urine from the kidney to the bladder) may lead to kidney damage. Fibroids that press on the bowels may cause constipation or hemorrhoids.

For some women, the pain of fibroids takes a more serious and disabling form. First, fibroids can cause unpleasant cramps. In addition, when a fibroid enlarges rapidly, acute, severe pain can result if there is degeneration or inflammation within the body of the fibroid itself. This is not an uncommon occurrence during pregnancy. Occasionally, a fibroid may twist on its stalk, a movement that can be extremely painful. A fibroid tumor that begins to prolapse downward through the cervix can cause dull, low-midline pelvic pain as well as pain during intercourse.

Infertility. Fibroids may be the cause in as many as 5 to 10 percent of infertility cases. Fibroids may inhibit implantation of the fertilized egg in the uterine lining by altering transport of the sperm, compressing the fallopian tube, or disrupting the lining of the uterus. In addition, fibroids may possibly cause spontaneous abortion during the first three months of pregnancy, either by distorting the uterine cavity or by altering the blood flow that would normally be needed to nourish the growing fetus. In any case, women with a history of infertility who wish to conceive should be carefully evaluated to determine the size and location of any preexisting fibroids.

Diagnosis of Fibroids

Fibroids can be diagnosed in several ways. Most commonly a preliminary diagnosis is made through an abdominal and pelvic examination. A uterus that contains fibroids will often feel enlarged, with an irregular contour. The uterus will probably have a hard, lumpy feel, although some fibroids may feel more soft and cystic. A diagnosis based on an abdominal and pelvic exam is correct about 85 percent of the time. Other conditions, such as an ovarian cancer or cyst, a pelvic inflammatory mass, a mass originating in the bowel, or even an early pregnancy, may occasionally be mistaken for a fibroid.

For further diagnosis, a pelvic ultrasound can be done. This is a visualization technique to identify lesions by their shape and density. Fibroids have specific visual characteristics on ultrasound that differentiate them from cysts and other structures. Tests, such as the intravenous pyelogram and barium enema, are imaging techniques used for the bowel and urinary tract. A blood count, urinalysis, and checks for blood in bowel movements may also be done when a physician undertakes a thorough evaluation of the pelvic mass.

When bleeding is the main symptom of a possible fibroid, the physician may take a tissue sample of the uterine lining or endometrium for diagnostic purposes. This is usually done in the physician's office through either an endometrial biopsy (which uses a small sampling device) or a D&C (which uses larger tools). The D&C also allows the physician to actually feel the irregularity of the endometrial surface typical of fibroid tumors. Once a definitive diagnosis of the fibroid is made, effective treatment can be instituted to alleviate the symptoms, promote regression of the tumor, and prevent more from forming. For details, refer to the treatment sections of this book.

Risk Factors for Fibroids

- Pregnancy

- Being premenopausal

- Use of high-dose estrogen birth control pills

- Anovulatory cycles

- Use of estrogen replacement therapy in postmenopausal women with preexisting fibroids

- Endometrial hyperplasia

- Obesity

- Family members with fibroids

- High-stress diet, with excessive use of alcohol, fat, red meat, dairy products, chocolate, sugar

- Lack of B vitamins

- Significant emotional or physical stress

Symptoms of Fibroids

- Heavy menstrual bleeding

- Irregular menstrual bleeding and spotting

- Pelvic pressure and pain

- Urinary frequency and urgency

- Constipation and hemorrhoids

- Infertility

- Loss of pregnancies

2

What Is Endometriosis?

$\mathcal{E}$ndometriosis refers to the condition in which cells comprising the lining of the uterus, called the endometrium, break away and grow outside the uterine cavity, implanting themselves in the pelvis. These implants can occur in many locations within the pelvis, including the ovaries, ligaments of the uterus, cervix, appendix, bowel, and bladder. Occasionally, these cells can even invade distant structures such as a lung or armpit. Like the regular lining of the uterus, these implants respond to hormonal stimulation and can cause bleeding in the pelvic cavity. Unlike normal menstrual bleeding, implant bleeding cannot leave the body through the vaginal opening during menstruation. Instead, blood from the endometrial implants remains trapped in the pelvis where it can cause inflammation, cysts, scar tissue, and other structural damage to the many tissues and organs in this area.

The endometrial implants can assume a variety of shapes and colors. They can include lesions that are tiny pinpoint areas of bleeding; white opaque plaques; or small lesions, rust or dark brown in color, that are described as "mulberry" or "raspberry" in appearance. Some medical textbooks describe these dark areas as looking like "powder burns." Fibrous tissue often grows around these lesions, giving them a puckered appearance. In more advanced cases, adhesions (scar tissue) develop around the implants. The scar tissue can be so dense that it obliterates the normal pelvic structures. Endometrial implants on the ovary can form cysts; these cysts are often called "chocolate cysts" because they are filled with a thick, dark brown fluid that is actually old blood. The inflammatory changes, scarring, and tissue damage associated with endometrial implants can destroy and distort the normal pelvic tissues in a way that causes significant problems for affected women.

Endometriosis is considered an important gynecological problem because it can cause chronic pain and discomfort in younger women during their prime reproductive years. In fact, it is found primarily in menstruating women from age 20 to 45, with its peak incidence in the thirties and forties. It is not, however, limited to this age group; endometriosis can be found in teenagers and even occasionally in postmenopausal women, since the estrogen used in hormone replacement therapy can reactivate the endometrial implants. Endometriosis is a relatively common problem, affecting as many as five million American women (or 7 to 15 percent of the female population). It is a major cause of chronic pain and severe menstrual cramps in younger women, affecting over 50 percent of those in their teens. The pelvic damage caused by endometriosis can also hamper childbearing. In fact, 20 to 66 percent of women with endometriosis experience infertility, a finding based on medical research and clinical studies. To better understand what causes this crippling problem, let's look at the normal menstrual cycle. This will make it easier to understand the changes in the normal process that can occur and lead to the development of endometriosis.

The Normal Menstrual Cycle

Each month women in their fertile years (before the onset of menopause, age 45 to 50) go through menstruation. Menstruation refers to the shedding of the uterine lining, or endometrium. Each month the uterus prepares a thick, blood-rich cushion to nourish and house a fertilized egg. If pregnancy doesn't occur and the egg doesn't implant in the uterus, then the body doesn't need this extra buildup of the uterine lining. The uterus cleanses itself by releasing the extra blood and tissue so that a fresh buildup can occur all over again the following month, in case a pregnancy does occur.

The mechanism that regulates the buildup and shedding of the uterine lining is controlled by fluctuations in hormonal levels. It begins each month when follicle-stimulating hormones (FSH) and luteinizing hormones (LH) are released from the pituitary, a gland located at the base of the brain. Once FSH and LH are released into the bloodstream, their destination is the ovaries. The ovaries hold all the eggs a woman will ever have, in an inactive form called follicles. During each cycle, the FSH and LH from the pituitary gland cause the follicles to ripen; normally, one egg is released for possible fertilization. As part of this process, the follicles begin to produce the hormones estrogen and progesterone. Estrogen reaches its peak during the first half of the cycle as the newly released egg is maturing. Progesterone output begins after midcycle when ovulation (the production of a mature egg cell) has occurred.

Besides preparing the egg for fertilization, estrogen and progesterone stimulate the lining of the uterus. During the first two weeks following menstruation, estrogen causes the uterine lining to gradually rebuild itself. The glands of the endometrium begin to grow long, and the lining thickens through an increase in the number of blood vessels as well as the production of a mesh of fibers that connect throughout the lining. By midcycle, the lining of the uterus has expanded three times in thickness and has a greatly increased blood supply.

After midcycle, usually around day 14, ovulation occurs. The egg is picked up by the fallopian tube and continues on to the uterus. The follicle that has produced the egg for that month (or graafian follicle) is further stimulated after midcycle by LH and changes into the yellow body, or *corpus luteum*. The *corpus luteum* secretes progesterone, which has further effects on the uterine lining, causing a coiling of the blood vessels of the endometrium. Also, the glands of the uterine lining become swollen and tortuous and secrete a thick mucous.

If the egg is fertilized, it will implant on the uterine wall and the *corpus luteum* will continue to secrete progesterone. If no fertilization occurs, the *corpus luteum* begins to deteriorate and the progesterone levels decrease. The lining of the uterus starts to break down and menstruation begins.

Besides estrogen and progesterone, the hormonelike prostaglandins also affect menstrual function by regulating the muscle tension of the uterus. Like progesterone, prostaglandin production is seen only during ovulatory menstrual cycles. Prostaglandin production increases during the second half of the cycle, peaking toward the end of the cycle with the onset of menstruation. Prostaglandins are found in many tissues in the body besides the uterus, including the gastrointestinal tract and blood vessels. All prostaglandins affect muscle tension, with some promoting smooth muscle relaxation while others trigger smooth muscle contraction.

Prostaglandins are derived from fatty acids in the diet. The series-two prostaglandins (specifically the E_2 and F_2 Alpha) that trigger muscle contractions are derived from animal fat—meat, dairy products, and eggs. The beneficial muscle-relaxant series-one and series-three prostaglandins are derived from vegetable and fish sources of fatty acids. These fatty acids, called linoleic acid and linolenic acid, are found predominantly in raw seeds and nuts, such as flax seed or pumpkin seed, and certain fish, such as trout, mackerel, and salmon. Thus, how we eat can determine which hormonal pathway we travel—toward muscle tension or muscle relaxation. This is a good example of how our food selection can determine our state of health.

Causes of Endometriosis

Medical research has not pinpointed one specific factor that initiates endometriosis. Instead, a variety of mechanical, hormonal, and immunological triggers may predispose women to developing this complex disease. The most likely theories about the cause of endometriosis are explained in the following paragraphs.

Theory: Menstrual Backup (Retrograde Menstruation). This theory, first proposed in 1921 by a researcher named John A. Simpson, suggests that endometriosis is caused by the backing up of pieces of the uterine lining, or endometrium, during menstruation. That is, instead of exiting through the vagina as part of the menstrual flow, some tissue backs up through the fallopian tubes and into the pelvic cavity. In the pelvis, these pieces of tissue implant onto pelvic organs such as the ovary and bowel. The tissue continues to function as the normal uterine lining would, responding to the cyclical hormonal output from the endocrine glands and bleeding on a monthly basis into the pelvic cavity.

This theory has had support from research done on animals such as monkeys, rabbits, and rats; when endometrial tissue was implanted into their pelvic cavities, the development of endometriosis followed. However, research on women, performed by doing laparoscopies (a surgical technique allowing visualization of the pelvis) during their menstrual periods, has shown that almost all women push blood through their fallopian tubes into the pelvic cavity during menstruation. Some researchers have suggested that this tendency is more pronounced in women whose uteruses are tipped backward, or retroverted. Other physicians have suggested that menstrual cramps caused by uterine spasm may predispose women toward developing endometriosis. None of these theories has been proven, and not all women develop endometriosis. Obviously, there are other factors that cause the endometrial tissue to implant and cause active disease.

Theory: Spread Through Blood Circulation and Lymph Glands. This theory was suggested by a researcher named J. Hilbran to explain why some endometrial implants occasionally are found as far away as a lung or armpit. Rather than invalidating the retrograde menstruation theory, Hilbran's theory simply offers alternate channels through which tissue of the uterine lining can spread to more distant sites. Blood and lymph circulate throughout the body and are natural pathways for the dissemination of endometrial tissue. This process, known as metastasis, is the same process by which cancer spreads in the body. However, once cancer or endometriosis spreads, the two conditions act entirely differently in their pattern of growth. While cancer consumes and destroys the host organ to which it attaches itself, the endometrial implants use the host as a place to embed themselves and grow.

Theory: Impaired Immune Function. As mentioned earlier, almost all women experience retrograde menstruation, but not all develop endometriosis. Some researchers have postulated that an impaired or altered immune response allows the endometrial implants to grow. Normally, the immune system protects us from disease-causing agents, including viruses, fungi, bacteria, and an array of other foreign invaders such as pollen, dust, pollutants, and chemicals. When the body encounters these agents, the immune system mounts a complex protective response. Our immune system also protects us against aberrant cells that arise within our own body, such as cancer cells, or possibly even aberrant endometrial tissue.

The immune system protects us by destroying these invaders and limiting the damage they can cause in the body, such as inflammation and swelling. The process involves the production of immune cells, including phagocytes, lymphocytes, antibodies, neutrophils, and macrophages. Each of these has a specific role in orchestrating the body's protection against invasion and disease; yet together these various cell types act as a supportive team.

When functioning efficiently, the immune system works beautifully to maintain good health. However, the immune system can become compromised and not perform its protective function effectively when our bodies are exposed to such environmental stresses as the excessive use of alcohol, recreational drugs, cigarettes, poor nutritional habits (with diets that are high in fat, sugar, and caffeinated beverages), and severe emotional upset.

Researchers have theorized that women with endometriosis may have a compromised immune function and are thus unable to halt the spread of endometriosis and limit the damage it causes to the pelvic organs. It is possible that when the immune system is compromised, the endometrial implants are able to spread throughout the pelvic region much more aggressively and are more likely to cause tissue damage, such as inflammation and scarring. This spread would normally be held in check by healthy immune function. Though research on this issue has not been conclusive, it is possible that compromised immune system function plays a role in the development and spread of this condition.

Risk Factors That Increase the Likelihood of Endometriosis

Whatever the cause of endometriosis, a number of factors can predispose a woman toward developing this problem. Though endometriosis can occur in women of any type or background during their active reproductive years, it does seem to occur more frequently in high-achieving career women who suffer from significant personal and career stress. Significant stress can disrupt the delicate hormonal balance in women, as well as weaken immune function, which can allow endometrial implants to grow and spread. Childlessness is also a risk factor for endometriosis and, in fact, pregnancy does seem to offer protection against developing the symptoms of this disease. This may be in part because women with multiple pregnancies have fewer menstrual cycles than do childless women, and thus have far less stimulation of the implants by the normal monthly hormonal fluctuations.

Endometriosis occurs primarily in Caucasian women, although many cases are found among women of Asian and African heritage and those of other ethnic and racial backgrounds. A familial predisposition to endometriosis seems to exist, and 8 to 10 percent of patients with endometriosis have mothers or sisters similarly afflicted. Women who suffer from recurrent stress to the immune system, such as chronic infections, may also be more prone to the development and spread of endometriosis. Weakened immune systems may be unable to control the proliferation of the implants as well as the inflammation and scarring that they cause in the pelvic area.

As mentioned earlier, the endometrial implants are stimulated by estrogen. As with fibroids, the excessive use of any food that elevates estrogen levels is a risk factor for worsening the spread and symptoms of endometriosis. The liver controls the levels of estrogen circulating through the body. It is responsible for deactivating estrogen chemically so that it can be excreted from the body. If the liver is unable to carry out this task efficiently because of a diet high in alcohol, fat, dairy products, red meat, sugar, and chocolate, estrogen levels can become elevated and worsen endometriosis. To deactivate estrogen, the liver also needs sufficient levels of certain B-complex vitamins, so a vitamin B deficiency can exacerbate the problem. Even obesity can contribute to endometriosis because overweight women tend to produce higher levels of estrogen.

The use of estrogen therapy is contraindicated for women with endometriosis. Such women should not be given estrogen-dominant birth control pills, and estrogen replacement therapy should be used very cautiously during the postmenopausal period. Otherwise, women are at risk of restimulating the implants, which often regress after menopause when estrogen levels decline.

In summary, many of the factors that predispose women to the spread of endometriosis can be modified and even eliminated through changes in lifestyle. This is true even for women whose racial, ethnic, and family background would put them in a higher risk category. The lifestyle modifications that can help eliminate endometriosis are discussed in the self-help section of this book.

Symptoms of Endometriosis

Endometriosis can present with a wide variety of symptoms. The types of symptoms and degree of severity depend on where the implants are located. Interestingly, 30 percent of women with endometriosis experience no symptoms at all and find out only incidentally that they have this problem. Typically this happens if the implants are located away from nerves and other sensitive structures within the pelvis. The other 70 percent of affected women can find endometriosis quite disabling, experiencing severe and recurrent symptoms. The most common symptoms found in women with endometriosis are described in the following paragraphs.

Menstrual Cramps and Pain. Approximately 60 percent of women with endometriosis suffer from progressively worsening menstrual cramps. Menstrual cramp problems caused by endometriosis often begin when women are in their twenties and thirties, although they can affect teenagers, also. Symptoms may occur for as long as two weeks premenstrually and can continue through menstruation. Cramps caused by endometriosis may be extremely painful and may not respond to the usual menstrual cramp medications, such as birth control pills or anti-inflammatory drugs.

The chronic pelvic pain caused by endometriosis may be due not only to stimulation of and bleeding from the implants, but also to the adhesions and pelvic scarring that inflammation in these implants causes over time. Many women with advanced endometriosis are discovered during surgery to have thick scar tissue that can deform or even obliterate the normal structure of the ovaries, ligaments, bowels, and other pelvic structures.

Some women with endometriosis also suffer from pain at ovulation (or mittelschmerz). Mid-month ovulation usually causes no pain in most women. However, in women with endometriosis, hormonal stimulation of the implants can cause a slight bleeding with subsequent irritation of nerve endings in the pelvic cavity. This can lead to pelvic pain lasting about two days.

Dyspareunia. This means pain on sexual intercourse. It can occur when there is endometrial invasion of the uterosacral ligaments or of a pouch located behind the uterus called the cul-de-sac, or pouch of Douglas. Implants growing in this area can push the uterus in a tilted-back position that doctors call retroversion. When the uterus is pulled backward out of its normal position, deep vaginal penetration during intercourse can become very painful. In fact, the pain can be so severe that sexual intercourse becomes too uncomfortable to participate in. Implants in the cul-de-sac can also be responsible for the low back pain that affects some women during menstruation.

Infertility. Endometriosis is a common cause of infertility. Medical studies have estimated that approximately 30 percent of women with endometriosis are unable to conceive. Endometriosis can cause infertility by scarring and obstructing the fallopian tubes so severely that the tubes cannot pick up the egg, or by scarring the ovaries so extensively that ovulation is prevented. In the general population, approximately 10 percent of women are estimated to be infertile. For women who have never been pregnant and still want to conceive and bear a child, this may be one of the more difficult emotional aspects surrounding endometriosis. Accomplishing a successful pregnancy may require long-term medical care, and even this effort does not always succeed.

Medical studies have found, not surprisingly, that the milder the case, the more likely a woman is to become pregnant after treatment of the endometriosis. For example, in one study done using Danazol (a common hormonal therapy for endometriosis, discussed further in Chapter 12), women with milder cases had more than twice the pregnancy rate of those with severe disease. Specifically among women with mild cases of disease, this meant an 83 percent success rate versus a 37 percent success rate within the first year of stopping drug therapy. Still the news is good for women in all stages of the disease, as fertility is a possible and achievable goal for a number of women with endometriosis-related infertility.

Abnormal Bleeding. Abnormal bleeding, including premenstrual spotting as well as excessive menstrual flow, occurs in approximately one-third of all women with endometriosis. In some cases of endometriosis, the menstrual cycles may also be irregular. Bleeding abnormalities in women with endometriosis may be due to lack of ovulation. In anovulatory cycles, progesterone is not secreted. Progesterone has an important effect on the uterine lining during the normal menstrual cycle and helps to limit the amount of blood flow. When progesterone is missing, blood flow can be excessive. When excessive bleeding or spotting happens frequently, iron-deficiency anemia may occur. Women with anemia due to excessive bleeding may find that their energy levels drop and that they lose stamina and endurance, in addition to the other symptoms of endometriosis.

Rectal and Bladder Involvement. When endometrial implants invade the small intestine or colon, unpleasant symptoms may result. Endometrial implants that invade the bowel can cause constipation, painful bowel movements, and rectal bleeding. Since hemorrhoids or even cancer can cause similar symptoms, all symptoms that might be caused by bowel invasion need to be carefully evaluated by a physician. Invasion of the small intestine by endometriosis can cause abdominal swelling, pain, and vomiting.

Occasionally, endometriosis will invade the bladder and cause symptoms similar to urinary tract infections with urinary frequency, pain on urination, urinary retention, and blood in the urine during menstruation.

Endometrial Cysts. These cysts, also called "chocolate cysts," tend to be deep brown in color, and are filled with old blood and endometrial cells. They can vary greatly in size, ranging from quite small to larger than a grapefruit. They tend to grow fast and even leak blood, which causes much pain. They can also rupture and present with symptoms much like acute appendicitis, a surgical emergency.

In summary, symptoms such as menstrual cramps and pain, pain on sexual intercourse, infertility, abnormal bleeding, blood and bladder symptoms, and endometrial cysts can be seen in varying degrees in women with endometriosis. How severe the symptoms are depend on the site of the implants and determine how aggressive the medical treatment needs to be to help relieve the symptoms and control the underlying process of endometriosis.

Diagnosis of Endometriosis

Physical signs of endometriosis can be noted during a pelvic exam by a gynecologist. Often, the uterus is fixed and not freely mobile; it can also be retroverted, or tilted backward. Endometrial, or chocolate cysts, may be large and easy to feel. Patients may complain of pelvic tenderness during the examination because of endometrial implants located in the pelvic region. Endometrial implants located in the uterosacral ligaments will feel nodular and shotty (hard and round, like a shot pellet) on examination. Tenderness is particularly noted at the time of menstruation.

For a definitive diagnosis of endometriosis, a laparoscopy is usually necessary. The laparoscope is a visualization device shaped like a thin tube. The device is inserted through a small abdominal incision. Gas is introduced into the abdomen to move the organs apart for better visualization of any disease process. This also allows the physician to see the ovaries and fallopian tubes. Laparoscopy enables the physician to see any lesions that have the typical appearance of endometriosis implants; puckered "powder burn" lesions, red lesions, and blueberry spots may commonly be seen, as well as white scar tissue, or adhesions, and chocolate ovarian cysts. Laparoscopy can also be used to determine if fertilization is impaired by the implants. By infusing a bluish colored dye through the fallopian tubes, the degree of openness (or patency) of the tubes can be evaluated. This is important for women who wish to become pregnant and for whom possible infertility caused by endometriosis is an issue.

Surgical treatment can usually be initiated at the time of laparoscopy. Adhesions and implants can be dissolved with a laser or by electrocauterization. However, there are women with endometriosis for whom laparoscopy is not advisable. These include patients with extensive endometriosis, massive scarring, or implants that have invaded deep into the ovaries, urinary tract, or bowels. These patients will often require more extensive surgery.

A similar technique called culdoscopy may also be performed. Culdoscopy was a more common diagnostic tool before the introduction of laparoscopy, which has superseded it in recent years. Unlike laparoscopy, culdoscopy must be done through an incision in the vaginal wall. A periscopelike instrument is introduced through this incision and allows a view of the uterus, ovaries, and fallopian tubes. A woman must be placed in an awkward position for the exam, which should be done under a local anesthetic. The intestines tend to fall forward with this exam, so the area behind the uterus is better visualized. However, this technique involves a somewhat higher risk of infection than laparoscopy, and it allows a more limited range of procedures to be performed.

Other imaging techniques may give additional clues to the locations of the endometrial implants. Ultrasound is a noninvasive technique that allows visualization of pelvic structures such as the uterus and ovaries by bouncing high-frequency sound waves off these solid masses. The waves bounce back in patterns that appear as pictures on a screen. The technique is particularly helpful in diagnosing chocolate ovarian cysts and fibroid tumors. In women with symptoms such as urinary frequency, blood in the urine at menstruation, and bladder pain, all of which suggest endometrial invasion of the bladder wall, specific X-rays of the genitourinary tract may be necessary.

Imaging of the genitourinary tract may be done with cystoscopy. In cystoscopy, a visualizing scope is inserted through the urethra into the bladder. Blockage or invasion of the urethra and bladder can be seen with this device. An intravenous pyelogram, which targets the kidneys, requires injecting dye into a vein. When the dye travels to the kidneys, X-rays are taken. This technique reveals an endometrial invasion of the kidneys as a telltale indentation. However, this technique does not specifically allow a diagnosis of endometriosis to be made, because other conditions, such as cancer, can also invade kidney tissue. In this case, a kidney biopsy may be necessary for a definitive diagnosis. Finally, an X-ray called a barium enema may help to better visualize endometrial growths in the intestines. A chalky, opaque liquid is passed through the colon and allows any growths or deformities to be seen by X-rays. A physician may request that a woman with suspected endometriosis do this procedure twice—once in the first half of the menstrual cycle and again during menstruation—to look for changes in the size of possible endometrial lesions due to hormonal fluctuations.

As you can see, a variety of techniques can help the physician differentiate endometriosis from menstrual cramps, ovarian cysts, pelvic infections, and a host of other symptoms. With accurate diagnosis of the exact locations of the implants, therapy can be targeted most effectively in the effort to combat this difficult disease.

Symptoms of Endometriosis

- Menstrual pain and cramps

- Pain at ovulation (mittelschmerz)

- Pelvic pain

- Low back pain

- Painful intercourse

- Infertility

- Excessive menstrual bleeding

- Premenstrual spotting

- Menstrual irregularity

- Constipation, painful bowel movements

- Rectal bleeding (especially with menstruation)

- Abdominal pain, swelling, vomiting

- Urinary frequency, pain on urination

- Blood in the urine during menstruation

Risk Factors for Endometriosis

- Childlessness

- High degree of personal and/or career stress

- Caucasian background

- Family members with endometriosis

- Immune system stress, such as chronic infections

- Use of estrogen-dominant birth control pills

- Use of estrogen replacement therapy

- Excessive use of alcohol, fat, dairy products, red meat, sugar, chocolate

- Lack of B vitamins

- Obesity

Evaluating
Your Symptoms

✦　　✦　　✦

3

The Fibroids & Endometriosis Workbook

 $\mathcal{A}$n important part of your self-help program is your personal evaluation of the fibroid or endometriosis problem for which you are seeking solutions. I have developed this workbook to help you evaluate your symptoms and identify your risk factors that can contribute to both fibroids and endometriosis.

First, begin to fill out the monthly calendar of fibroid and endometriosis symptoms, starting today. If you recall your symptoms for the past month, chart these symptoms as well. The calendar will enable you to record the types of symptoms you have, as well as evaluate their severity. This will make it easier for you to pick the appropriate treatments for symptom relief. Then, as you follow the program, you can keep using the monthly calendars (a year's worth have been included) to check your progress.

After you've started the calendar, turn to the risk factor and lifestyle evaluations that follow the calendar section. They will help you assess specific areas of your life—diet, exercise, stress— to see which of your habit patterns may be contributing to your health problems. I have found that lifestyle habits significantly affect the symptoms of fibroids and endometriosis. By filling out the lifestyle evaluation forms, you can easily recognize your weak areas. When you've completed these evaluations, you will be ready to go on to the self-help chapters that follow and begin planning and initiating your personal treatment program.

Besides helping you plan your own program, these charts can be useful when you discuss your situation with your physician. The information contained in these charts about your symptoms, lifestyle habits, and possible risk factors can help your physician assess the severity of your problem as well as determine the need for medical intervention. I have personally found it very helpful when my patients share these charts with me.

Monthly Calendar of Fibroid and Endometriosis Symptoms

Grade your symptoms as you experience them each month:
○ None ✓ Mild ◗ Moderate ▲ Severe

Day of month Symptom	1	2	3	4	5	6	7	8	9	10
Heavy menstrual bleeding										
Spotting										
Spasmodic/stabbing menstrual cramps and pain										
Low back pain										
Premenstrual pain up to two weeks prior to onset										
Pain in inner thighs										
Abdominal tenderness										
Nausea and vomiting										
Diarrhea										
Constipation										
Bloating										
Hot and cold										
Faintness, dizziness										
Fatigue										
Headaches										
Pain at midcycle (mittleschmerz)										
Pain during or after intercourse										
Rectal bleeding										
Urinary frequency										
Blood in the urine										

Month 1 _____

11	12	13	14	15	16	17	18	19	20	21	22	23	24	25	26	27	28	29	30	31

Monthly Calendar of Fibroid and Endometriosis Symptoms

Grade your symptoms as you experience them each month:
O None   ✓ Mild   ◗ Moderate   ▲ Severe

Day of month **Symptom**	1	2	3	4	5	6	7	8	9	10
Heavy menstrual bleeding										
Spotting										
Spasmodic/stabbing menstrual cramps and pain										
Low back pain										
Premenstrual pain up to two weeks prior to onset										
Pain in inner thighs										
Abdominal tenderness										
Nausea and vomiting										
Diarrhea										
Constipation										
Bloating										
Hot and cold										
Faintness, dizziness										
Fatigue										
Headaches										
Pain at midcycle (mittleschmerz)										
Pain during or after intercourse										
Rectal bleeding										
Urinary frequency										
Blood in the urine										

Month 2 _____

11	12	13	14	15	16	17	18	19	20	21	22	23	24	25	26	27	28	29	30	31

Monthly Calendar of Fibroid and Endometriosis Symptoms

Grade your symptoms as you experience them each month:
◯ None   ✓ Mild   ▶ Moderate   ▲ Severe

Day of month Symptom	1	2	3	4	5	6	7	8	9	10
Heavy menstrual bleeding										
Spotting										
Spasmodic/stabbing menstrual cramps and pain										
Low back pain										
Premenstrual pain up to two weeks prior to onset										
Pain in inner thighs										
Abdominal tenderness										
Nausea and vomiting										
Diarrhea										
Constipation										
Bloating										
Hot and cold										
Faintness, dizziness										
Fatigue										
Headaches										
Pain at midcycle (mittleschmerz)										
Pain during or after intercourse										
Rectal bleeding										
Urinary frequency										
Blood in the urine										

Month 3 _____

11	12	13	14	15	16	17	18	19	20	21	22	23	24	25	26	27	28	29	30	31

Monthly Calendar of Fibroid and Endometriosis Symptoms

Grade your symptoms as you experience them each month:

○ None   ✓ Mild   ◗ Moderate   ▲ Severe

Day of month Symptom	1	2	3	4	5	6	7	8	9	10
Heavy menstrual bleeding										
Spotting										
Spasmodic/stabbing menstrual cramps and pain										
Low back pain										
Premenstrual pain up to two weeks prior to onset										
Pain in inner thighs										
Abdominal tenderness										
Nausea and vomiting										
Diarrhea										
Constipation										
Bloating										
Hot and cold										
Faintness, dizziness										
Fatigue										
Headaches										
Pain at midcycle (mittleschmerz)										
Pain during or after intercourse										
Rectal bleeding										
Urinary frequency										
Blood in the urine										

Month 4 _____

11	12	13	14	15	16	17	18	19	20	21	22	23	24	25	26	27	28	29	30	31

Monthly Calendar of Fibroid and Endometriosis Symptoms

Grade your symptoms as you experience them each month:

○ None   ✓ Mild   ◗ Moderate   ▲ Severe

Day of month	1	2	3	4	5	6	7	8	9	10
Symptom										
Heavy menstrual bleeding										
Spotting										
Spasmodic/stabbing menstrual cramps and pain										
Low back pain										
Premenstrual pain up to two weeks prior to onset										
Pain in inner thighs										
Abdominal tenderness										
Nausea and vomiting										
Diarrhea										
Constipation										
Bloating										
Hot and cold										
Faintness, dizziness										
Fatigue										
Headaches										
Pain at midcycle (mittleschmerz)										
Pain during or after intercourse										
Rectal bleeding										
Urinary frequency										
Blood in the urine										

Month 5 _____

11	12	13	14	15	16	17	18	19	20	21	22	23	24	25	26	27	28	29	30	31

Monthly Calendar of Fibroid and Endometriosis Symptoms

Grade your symptoms as you experience them each month:

○ None   ✓ Mild   ◗ Moderate   ▲ Severe

Day of month **Symptom**	1	2	3	4	5	6	7	8	9	10
Heavy menstrual bleeding										
Spotting										
Spasmodic/stabbing menstrual cramps and pain										
Low back pain										
Premenstrual pain up to two weeks prior to onset										
Pain in inner thighs										
Abdominal tenderness										
Nausea and vomiting										
Diarrhea										
Constipation										
Bloating										
Hot and cold										
Faintness, dizziness										
Fatigue										
Headaches										
Pain at midcycle (mittleschmerz)										
Pain during or after intercourse										
Rectal bleeding										
Urinary frequency										
Blood in the urine										

Month 6 _____

11	12	13	14	15	16	17	18	19	20	21	22	23	24	25	26	27	28	29	30	31

Monthly Calendar of Fibroid and Endometriosis Symptoms

Grade your symptoms as you experience them each month:

○ None   ✓ Mild   ❯ Moderate   ▲ Severe

Day of month — Symptom	1	2	3	4	5	6	7	8	9	10
Heavy menstrual bleeding										
Spotting										
Spasmodic/stabbing menstrual cramps and pain										
Low back pain										
Premenstrual pain up to two weeks prior to onset										
Pain in inner thighs										
Abdominal tenderness										
Nausea and vomiting										
Diarrhea										
Constipation										
Bloating										
Hot and cold										
Faintness, dizziness										
Fatigue										
Headaches										
Pain at midcycle (mittleschmerz)										
Pain during or after intercourse										
Rectal bleeding										
Urinary frequency										
Blood in the urine										

Month 7 _____

11	12	13	14	15	16	17	18	19	20	21	22	23	24	25	26	27	28	29	30	31

Monthly Calendar of Fibroid and Endometriosis Symptoms

Grade your symptoms as you experience them each month:

○ None ✓ Mild ◗ Moderate ▲ Severe

Day of month Symptom	1	2	3	4	5	6	7	8	9	10
Heavy menstrual bleeding										
Spotting										
Spasmodic/stabbing menstrual cramps and pain										
Low back pain										
Premenstrual pain up to two weeks prior to onset										
Pain in inner thighs										
Abdominal tenderness										
Nausea and vomiting										
Diarrhea										
Constipation										
Bloating										
Hot and cold										
Faintness, dizziness										
Fatigue										
Headaches										
Pain at midcycle (mittleschmerz)										
Pain during or after intercourse										
Rectal bleeding										
Urinary frequency										
Blood in the urine										

Month 8 _____

11	12	13	14	15	16	17	18	19	20	21	22	23	24	25	26	27	28	29	30	31

Monthly Calendar of Fibroid and Endometriosis Symptoms

Grade your symptoms as you experience them each month:

○ None   ✓ Mild   ❱ Moderate   ▲ Severe

Day of month Symptom	1	2	3	4	5	6	7	8	9	10
Heavy menstrual bleeding										
Spotting										
Spasmodic/stabbing menstrual cramps and pain										
Low back pain										
Premenstrual pain up to two weeks prior to onset										
Pain in inner thighs										
Abdominal tenderness										
Nausea and vomiting										
Diarrhea										
Constipation										
Bloating										
Hot and cold										
Faintness, dizziness										
Fatigue										
Headaches										
Pain at midcycle (mittleschmerz)										
Pain during or after intercourse										
Rectal bleeding										
Urinary frequency										
Blood in the urine										

Month 9 _____

11	12	13	14	15	16	17	18	19	20	21	22	23	24	25	26	27	28	29	30	31

Monthly Calendar of Fibroid and Endometriosis Symptoms

Grade your symptoms as you experience them each month:
○ None ✓ Mild ◗ Moderate ▲ Severe

Day of month **Symptom**	1	2	3	4	5	6	7	8	9	10
Heavy menstrual bleeding										
Spotting										
Spasmodic/stabbing menstrual cramps and pain										
Low back pain										
Premenstrual pain up to two weeks prior to onset										
Pain in inner thighs										
Abdominal tenderness										
Nausea and vomiting										
Diarrhea										
Constipation										
Bloating										
Hot and cold										
Faintness, dizziness										
Fatigue										
Headaches										
Pain at midcycle (mittleschmerz)										
Pain during or after intercourse										
Rectal bleeding										
Urinary frequency										
Blood in the urine										

Month 10 _____

11	12	13	14	15	16	17	18	19	20	21	22	23	24	25	26	27	28	29	30	31

Monthly Calendar of Fibroid and Endometriosis Symptoms

Grade your symptoms as you experience them each month:

○ None ✓ Mild ▶ Moderate ▲ Severe

Day of month **Symptom**	1	2	3	4	5	6	7	8	9	10
Heavy menstrual bleeding										
Spotting										
Spasmodic/stabbing menstrual cramps and pain										
Low back pain										
Premenstrual pain up to two weeks prior to onset										
Pain in inner thighs										
Abdominal tenderness										
Nausea and vomiting										
Diarrhea										
Constipation										
Bloating										
Hot and cold										
Faintness, dizziness										
Fatigue										
Headaches										
Pain at midcycle (mittleschmerz)										
Pain during or after intercourse										
Rectal bleeding										
Urinary frequency										
Blood in the urine										

Month 11 _____

11	12	13	14	15	16	17	18	19	20	21	22	23	24	25	26	27	28	29	30	31

Monthly Calendar of Fibroid and Endometriosis Symptoms

Grade your symptoms as you experience them each month:
○ None ✓ Mild ▶ Moderate ▲ Severe

Day of month Symptom	1	2	3	4	5	6	7	8	9	10
Heavy menstrual bleeding										
Spotting										
Spasmodic/stabbing menstrual cramps and pain										
Low back pain										
Premenstrual pain up to two weeks prior to onset										
Pain in inner thighs										
Abdominal tenderness										
Nausea and vomiting										
Diarrhea										
Constipation										
Bloating										
Hot and cold										
Faintness, dizziness										
Fatigue										
Headaches										
Pain at midcycle (mittleschmerz)										
Pain during or after intercourse										
Rectal bleeding										
Urinary frequency										
Blood in the urine										

Month 12 _____

11	12	13	14	15	16	17	18	19	20	21	22	23	24	25	26	27	28	29	30	31

Risk Factors for Fibroids and Endometriosis

You are at higher risk of developing fibroids or endometriosis and suffering from symptoms caused by either of these problems if you have any of the following risk factors. Be sure to follow the nutritional, exercise, and stress management guidelines in the self-help section of this book if any of the related risk factors apply to you. Check each risk factor that applies to you.

Risk Factors

Career or working woman	___
High-stress life, combining work and child care	___
Age twenties through forties	___
Childlessness (endometriosis)	___
Multiple pregnancies (fibroids)	___
Tendency toward ovarian cysts that bleed (endometriosis)	___
Mothers or sisters with a history of endometriosis or fibroids	___
High levels of estrogen as determined by your physician, or use of estrogen-containing medication	___
High levels of prostaglandin hormones as determined by your physician	___
Repeated laparoscopies	___
Significant life stress	
Emotional distress that hampers well-being, anxiety, depression	___
Concurrent immune stress, recurrent or chronic infections, allergies	___
High dietary intake of meat, saturated fat, dairy products, alcohol, sugar, caffeine, salt, or chocolate	___
Lack of B vitamins	___
Lack of exercise	___

Eating Habits and
Fibroids or Endometriosis

All the foods in the shaded area of the following list are high-stress foods that can worsen the symptoms of both problems. If you eat many of these foods, or if you eat any of these foods frequently, your nutritional habits may be contributing significantly to your symptoms. Read the chapters on dietary principles and meal plans and recipes for further guidance on food selection.

All the foods from avocado to fish are high-nutrient, low-stress foods that may help to relieve or prevent fibroid and endometriosis symptoms. Include these foods frequently in your diet. If you are already eating many of these foods and few of the high-stress foods, chances are your nutritional habits are good, and food selection may not be a significant factor in worsening your fibroids or endometriosis. You may want to look carefully at the stress management and exercise chapters. The activities contained in these chapters may be very helpful in relieving your symptoms.

Eating Habits Checklist

Check the number of times you eat the following foods.

Foods That Increase Symptoms

Foods	Never	Once a month	Once a week	Twice a week +
Cow's milk				
Cow's cheese				
Butter				
Yogurt				
Eggs				
Chocolate				
Sugar				
Alcohol				
Wheat bread				
Wheat noodles				

Foods	Never	Once a month	Once a week	Twice a week +
Wheat-based flour				
Pastries				
Added salt				
Bouillon				
Commercial salad dressing				
Catsup				
Coffee				
Black tea				
Soft drinks				
Hot dogs				
Ham				
Bacon				
Beef				
Lamb				
Pork				

Foods That Decrease Symptoms

Avocado				
Beans				
Beets				
Broccoli				
Brussels sprouts				
Cabbage				
Carrots				
Celery				
Collard greens				
Cucumbers				
Eggplant				
Garlic				
Horseradish				
Kale				
Lettuce				

Foods	Never	Once a month	Once a week	Twice a week +
Mustard greens				
Okra				
Onions				
Parsnips				
Peas				
Potatoes				
Radishes				
Rutabagas				
Spinach				
Squash				
Sweet potatoes				
Tomatoes				
Turnips				
Turnip greens				
Yams				
Brown rice				
Millet				
Barley				
Oatmeal				
Buckwheat				
Rye				
Raw flax seeds				
Corn				
Raw pumpkin seeds				
Raw sesame seeds				
Raw sunflower seeds				
Raw almonds				
Raw filberts				
Raw pecans				
Raw walnuts				
Apples				
Bananas				

Foods	Never	Once a month	Once a week	Twice a week +
Berries				
Pears				
Seasonal fruits				
Corn oil				
Flax oil				
Olive oil				
Sesame oil				
Safflower oil				
Poultry				
Fish				

Exercise Habits and Fibroids or Endometriosis

Exercise helps prevent the pain and cramps related to fibroids or endometriosis by relaxing muscles and promoting better blood circulation and oxygenation to the pelvic area. Exercise can also help reduce stress and relieve anxiety and upset. If your total number of exercise periods per week is less than three, you will probably be prone to pain and cramp symptoms. See the chapters on the various kinds of exercise that can help relieve and prevent symptoms.

If you are exercising more than three times a week, keep doing your exercises; they are probably making your symptoms less severe. You may want to add specific corrective exercises to your present regime, choosing them to fit your individual symptoms. You will find many options available in the chapters on exercise, yoga, and acupressure massage.

Exercise Checklist

Check the frequency with which you do any of the following activities.

Activity	Never	Once a month	Once a week	Twice a week +
Walking				
Running				
Dancing				
Swimming				
Bicycling				
Tennis				
Stretching				
Yoga				

Stress and Fibroids or Endometriosis

Checking many items in the first third of the following scale indicates major life stress and a possible vulnerability to serious illness. In other words, the more items checked in the first third, the higher your stress quotient. *Do everything possible to manage your stress in a healthy way.* Eat the foods that provide a high-nutrient/low-stress diet, exercise on a regular basis, and learn the methods for managing stress given in the chapters on stress reduction and deep breathing.

If you have checked fewer items, you are probably at low risk of illness caused by stress. But because stresses too small to figure in this evaluation may also play a part in worsening your fibroid and endometriosis symptoms, you would still benefit from practicing the methods outlined in the chapter on stress reduction. Stress management is very important in helping you gain control over your level of muscle tension.

Major Stress Evaluation

Check each stressful event that applies to you.

Life Events

___ Death of spouse or close family member
___ Divorce from spouse
___ Death of a close friend

___ Legal separation from spouse

___ Loss of job

___ Radical loss of financial security

___ Major personal injury or illness (gynecologic or other cause)

___ Future surgery for gynecologic or other illness

___ Beginning a new marriage

___ Foreclosure of mortgage or loan

___ Lawsuit lodged against you

___ Marriage reconciliation

___ Change in health of a family member

___ Major trouble with boss or co-workers

___ Increase in responsibility—job or home

___ Learning you are pregnant

___ Difficulties with your sexual abilities

___ Gaining a new family member

___ Change to a different job

___ Increase in number of marital arguments

___ New loan or mortgage of more than $100,000

___ Son or daughter leaving home

___ Major disagreement with in-laws or friends

___ Recognition for outstanding achievements

___ Spouse begins or stops work

___ Begin or end education

___ Undergo a change in living conditions

___ Revise or alter your personal habits

___ Change in work hours or conditions

___ Change of residence

___ Change your school or major in school

___ Alterations in your recreational activities

___ Change in church or club activities

___ Change in social activities

___ Change in sleeping habits

___ Change in number of family get-togethers

_____ Diet or eating habits are changed
_____ You go on vacation
_____ The year-end holidays occur
_____ You commit a minor violation of the law

Major life stress can have a significant impact on the symptoms of fibroids and endometriosis as well as other health problems. It is helpful to assess your level of stress to see how it may be affecting your health. One popular tool is the Holmes and Rahe Social Readjustment Rating Scale, first published in 1967, which gives you a stress "score." The scale above is adapted for women and simply identifies major life events that cause stress.

Daily Stress Evaluation

This evaluation is a very important one for women with fibroids or endometriosis. Not all stresses have a major impact in our lives, as do death, divorce, or personal injury. Most of us are exposed to a multitude of small life stresses on a daily basis. The effects of these stresses are cumulative and can be a major factor in worsening fibroid- or endometriosis-related muscle tension and pain in the pelvic area. After completing the checklist, read over the day-to-day stress areas that you find difficult to handle. Becoming aware of them is the first step toward lessening their effects on your life. Methods for reducing them and helping your body to deal with them are given in Chapter 7.

Check each item that seems to apply to you.

Work

_____ **Too much responsibility.** You feel you have to push too hard to do your work. There are too many demands made of you. You feel very pressured by all of this responsibility. You worry about getting all your work done and doing it well.

_____ **Time urgency.** You worry about getting your work

done on time. You always feel rushed. It feels like there are not enough hours in the day to complete your work.

___ **Job instability.** You are concerned about losing your job. There are layoffs at your company. There is much insecurity and concern among your fellow employees about their job security.

___ **Job performance.** You don't feel that you are working up to your maximum capability due to outside pressures or stress. You are unhappy with your job performance and concerned about job security as a result.

___ **Difficulty getting along with co-workers and boss.** Your boss is too picky and critical. Your boss demands too much. You must work closely with co-workers who are difficult to get along with.

___ **Understimulation.** Work is boring. The lack of stimulation makes you tired. You wish you were somewhere else.

___ **Uncomfortable physical plant.** Lights are too bright or too dim; noises are too loud. You're exposed to noxious fumes or chemicals. There is too much activity going on around you, making it difficult to concentrate.

Spouse or Significant Other

___ **Hostile communication.** There is too much negative emotion and drama. You are always upset and angry. There is not enough peace and quiet.

___ **Not enough communication.** There is not enough discussion of feelings or issues. You both tend to hold in your feelings. You feel that an emotional bond is lacking between you.

___ **Discrepancy in communication.** One person talks about feelings too much, the other person too little.

___ **Affection.** You do not feel you receive enough affection. There is not enough holding, touching, and loving in your relationship. Or, you are made uncomfortable by your partner's demands.

___ **Sexuality.** There is not enough sexual intimacy. You feel deprived by your partner. Or, your partner demands sexual relations too often. You feel pressured.

___ **Children.** They make too much noise. They make too many demands on your time. They are hard to discipline.

___ **Organization.** Home is poorly organized. It always seems messy; chores are half-finished.

___ **Time.** There is too much to do in the home and never enough time to get it all done.

___ **Responsibility.** You need more help. There are too many demands on your time and energy.

Your Emotional State

___ **Too much anxiety.** You worry too much about every little thing. You constantly worry about what can go wrong in your life.

___ **Victimization.** Everyone is taking advantage of you or wants to hurt you.

___ **Poor self-image.** You don't like yourself enough. You are always finding fault with yourself.

___ **Too critical.** You are always finding fault with others. You always look at what is wrong with other people rather than seeing their virtues.

___ **Inability to relax.** You are always wound up. It is difficult for you to relax. You are tense and restless.

___ **Not enough self-renewal.** You don't play enough or take enough time off to relax and have fun. Life isn't fun and enjoyable as a result.

___ **Feeling of depression.** You feel blue, isolated, and tearful. You feel a sense of self-blame and hopelessness. Fatigue and low energy are problems.

___ **Too angry.** Small life issues seem to upset you unduly. You find yourself becoming angry and irritable with your husband, children, or clients.

How Stress Affects Your Body

The following checklist should help you become aware of where stress localizes in your body. Each woman accumulates stress in a different way, tensing and contracting different sets of muscles in a pattern unique to her. Storing tension in the low back and pelvic area can worsen cramps, while storing it in the neck can cause headaches. This accumulation also increases your level of fatigue and lowers your energy and vitality.

Check the places where tension most commonly localizes in your body.

___ Low back
___ Pelvic area
___ Stomach muscles
___ Thighs and calves
___ Chest
___ Shoulders

_____ Arms

_____ Neck and throat

_____ Headache

_____ Grinding teeth

_____ Eyestrain

It is important to be aware of where you store tension. When you feel tension building up in these areas, begin deep breathing (Chapter 8) or use one of the stress-reduction techniques given in Chapter 7. Often, these techniques will help release muscle tension rapidly.

Finding
the Solution

✦　✦　✦

4

Dietary Principles for Relief of Fibroids & Endometriosis

*I*cannot emphasize too strongly the importance of good dietary habits for women beginning a fibroid and endometriosis treatment program. After years of working with thousands of women patients, including many with these problems, I have found that no therapy can be fully effective without including beneficial dietary changes as part of the treatment plan. The best therapeutic program can be subverted by a diet full of saturated fat, sugar, salt, caffeine, alcohol, and other high-stress food items. While many of these ingredients are found in the commonly eaten American "fast foods" and "junk foods," they are also found in foods that are considered staples.

Many women eat a diet they mistakenly think is healthy, not realizing that their food selection is actually worsening their symptoms. Luckily, the list of foods that help relieve and prevent fibroids and endometriosis is a long one. Once you shift to a diet of these more healthful foods, you will find that they are just as delicious, convenient, and easy to prepare as the foods you are eating now.

I discuss in this chapter both the foods to avoid and foods to emphasize for fibroids and endometriosis relief. The information on these foods is the result of almost two decades of work with women who have come to me with these problems and have had significant relief of their symptoms. I have been very impressed by how many women with fibroids and endometriosis have reported a noticeable decrease in heavy bleeding as well as pain and discomfort level within one or two menstrual cycles after starting my program. Besides the specific benefits these dietary principles will have on your cramps, they will also aid your general health and well-being. Many women have reported that they have more energy and a greater sense of well-being than they have had in years. Often they tell me that symptoms they never associated with their menstrual bleeding and cramps, such as allergies and generally poor digestive function, have cleared up as well. I hope the same great results happen for you, too!

Foods That Help Treat or Prevent Fibroids & Endometriosis

You should emphasize the following foods in your diet. They will provide the range of nutrients that you need to help balance your hormones, reduce your estrogen level, decrease cramping and inflammation, and generally improve your physical and mental well-being. Even though fibroid and endometriosis symptoms are worse during the second half of the menstrual cycle, these healthful foods should form the mainstay of your diet throughout the entire month. A poorly chosen high-stress diet during your symptom-free time will increase the severity of your symptoms when menstruation starts.

Whole Grains. I strongly recommend the use of certain whole grains such as millet, buckwheat, oats, and rice. Many women also tolerate 100% rye well. Whole grains are excellent sources of vitamin B and vitamin E, both of which are critical for healthy hormonal balance and lowering excessive estrogen levels through their beneficial effect on both the liver and ovaries. The vitamin B and vitamin E content of whole grains also help combat the fatigue and depression that is often seen with the onset of menstruation.

Grains are excellent sources of magnesium, which helps reduce neuromuscular tension and thereby decreases menstrual cramps. They are also fairly high in calcium, which relaxes muscle contraction. In addition, they are excellent sources of potassium. Potassium has a diuretic effect on the body tissues and helps reduce bloating. Excessive fluid retention is one of the main causes of the congestive symptoms seen with cramps that are characterized by dull, aching pain.

While many whole grains are beneficial, women with severe fibroid and endometriosis symptoms may need to avoid whole wheat and even try a wheat-free diet. This probably comes as a surprise to you because wheat is a mainstay of the American diet. However, wheat contains a protein called gluten that is difficult to digest and can be highly allergenic. In a number of women patients who had fibroids or endometriosis coexisting with PMS symptoms, I have seen wheat worsen their fatigue, depression, bloating, constipation, diarrhea, and intestinal cramps. You may want to try a wheat-free diet to see if you feel better once wheat is eliminated. If you have more severe gluten intolerance or food allergies, you may want to eliminate oats and rye also, since they contain some gluten as well. You may find that you feel best eating buckwheat, corn, and rice.

Whole grains provide other benefits to fibroid or endometriosis sufferers. The fiber in whole grains absorbs estrogen and helps remove it from the body through bowel elimination. This benefit of whole grain fiber was reported in the 1980s in *The New England Journal of Medicine.* In this study, it was found that vegetarian women who eat a high fiber, low fat diet have lower blood estrogen levels than omnivorous women with low fiber diets. Fiber can also help decrease the congestive symptoms of cramps since it produces bulkier stools with a higher water content. This helps to eliminate excessive fluid from the body. In addition, they are excellent sources of protein, especially when combined with beans and peas. I strongly recommend vegetable sources of protein for women with these two problems, since such proteins are easily digestible.

Fiber may also be helpful in reducing the digestive symptoms that occur with fibroids or endometriosis. It has a normalizing effect on the bowel movements, helping to eliminate both constipation and diarrhea. Besides removing excessive estrogen and water from the body, whole grains help to bind dietary fat and eliminate it from the body as well as help to lower cholesterol. Oat and rice bran are particularly good for this purpose. Because cancers of the breast, uterus, ovaries, and colon are linked to a diet high in animal fats, the use of whole grains may have a protective effect in preventing the development of these diseases.

Legumes. The best legumes to eat for relief of fibroid and endometriosis symptoms are soybeans. This includes many soy products like tofu, tempeh, boiled soy beans, and foods made from soy flour, like pasta. Substitute dairy products like soy yogurt are also available in health food stores.

The abundant use of soybeans in the diet actually help regulate and lower estrogen levels in the body. This is because soy is a rich source of natural plant estrogens, called bioflavonoids. The bioflavonoids found in soybeans have a chemical structure similar to estrogen, yet is much weaker in potency than the estrogen made by our bodies. (Bioflavonoids have only 1/50,000 the potency of synthetic estrogen.) Utilized in the diet, bioflavonoids actually compete with our body's own estrogen for binding to the estrogen receptors of our cells. Thus the weaker bioflavonoids can actually replace our own estrogen when binding to the uterus, breasts and other estrogen-sensitive tissue. Bioflavonoids can also help lower estrogen levels in the body by actually interfering with estrogen production.

The use of soy foods or the use of the bioflavonoids in a purified form have been found to help reduce bleeding problems in premenopausal women with fibroid tumors or who are not ovulating. Soybean use reduces the risk of breast cancer and can even help relieve menopausal symptoms in women who are estrogen deficient by adding an additional dietary source of this important hormone.

Beans and peas are excellent sources of calcium, magnesium, and potassium. I highly recommend their dietary use for fibroid and endometriosis relief. Particularly good choices include tofu, black beans, pinto beans, kidney beans, chickpeas, lentils, lima beans, and soybeans. These foods are also high in iron and tend to be good sources of copper and zinc; women with fibroids and endometriosis who suffer from heavy bleeding are often deficient in these minerals, particularly iron. Legumes are very high in vitamin B complex and vitamin B_6, necessary nutrients for healthy liver function, reducing excess estrogen levels, and prevention of cramps and menstrual fatigue. They are also excellent sources of protein and can be used as substitutes for meat at many meals; legumes provide all the essential amino acids when eaten with grains. Good examples of grain and legume combinations include meals such as beans and rice, or corn bread and split pea soup.

Like grains, legumes are a good source of fiber and can help normalize bowel function and lower cholesterol. They digest slowly and can help to regulate the blood sugar level, a trait they share with whole grains. As a result, they are an excellent food for women with diabetes or blood sugar imbalances. Some women find that gas is a problem when they eat beans. You can minimize gas by using digestive enzymes, adding powdered ginger to beans as they are cooking, and of course, eating beans in small quantities.

Vegetables. These are outstanding foods for relief of fibroid and endometriosis symptoms of all types. Many vegetables are high in calcium, magnesium, and potassium, which help to relieve and prevent the spasmodic symptoms of cramps. Besides helping relax tense, irritable muscles, these minerals help calm and relax the emotions, too. Both calcium and magnesium act as natural tranquilizers, a real benefit for women suffering from menstrual pain, discomfort, and irritability. The potassium content of vegetables helps to relieve the symptoms of menstrual congestion by reducing fluid retention and bloating. Some of the best sources for these minerals include Swiss chard, spinach, broccoli, beet greens, mustard greens, sweet potatoes, kale, potatoes, green peas, and green beans. These vegetables are also high in iron, which may help reduce bleeding and cramps.

Many vegetables are high in vitamin C, which helps decrease capillary fragility and facilitate the flow of essential nutrients into the tight muscles as well as the flow of waste products out. Decreased capillary fragility also means a reduction in the heavy menstrual bleeding commonly seen with fibroids and endometriosis. Vitamin C is an important antistress vitamin because it is needed for healthy adrenal hormonal production (the adrenals are important glands that help the body deal with stress). Vitamin C is also important for immune function and wound healing. Because of these properties, vitamin C may help limit the scarring and inflammation caused in the pelvis by the endometrial implants. Its anti-infectious properties may reduce the tendency toward bladder and vaginal infections. Vegetables high in vitamin C include brussels sprouts, broccoli, cauliflower, kale, peppers, parsley, peas, tomatoes, and potatoes.

Fruits. Fruits also contain a wide range of nutrients that can benefit menstrual cramps. Like many vegetables, fruits are an excellent source of vitamin C and bioflavonoids. Both of these nutrients prevent capillary fragility and reduce heavy menstrual flow. By strengthening blood vessels, they promote good blood circulation into the tense pelvic muscles. Almost all fruits contain some vitamin C, with the best sources being berries, oranges, grapefruits, and melons. These fruits are also good sources of bioflavonoids.

Bioflavonoids, interestingly enough, are also weakly estrogenic and antiestrogenic. This was first discovered many years ago when sheep grazing on certain types of clover showed estrogenic stimulation of the uterus. When analyzed chemically, however, these natural plant estrogens were found to be only 1/50,000 as potent as the levels used in drugs. Though bioflavonoids are weakly estrogenic themselves, they interfere with the production of estrogen by competing with estrogen precursors for binding sites on enzymes. Thus, bioflavonoids help to normalize the body's estrogen levels. They help elevate estrogen levels when they are too low, as in menopausal women, and help bring down excessive estrogen levels when they are too high, as may occur in women with fibroids and endometriosis.

This normalizing effect of the bioflavonoids has been shown in a variety of interesting studies. Bioflavonoids helped reduce the hot flashes and night sweats of menopause, and helped control heavy menstrual bleeding in conditions such as fibroid tumors and premenopause. Unlike drug levels of estrogen, the potency of the flavonoids is so weak that they do not appear to cause side effects.

Certain fruits are also excellent sources of calcium and magnesium; you can eat them often for your mineral needs. These include dried figs, raisins, blackberries, bananas, and oranges. Figs, raisins, and bananas are also exceptional sources of potassium, so should be eaten by women with fatigue and bloating. All fruits, in fact, are an excellent source of potassium. Eat fruits whole to take advantage of their high fiber content. This fiber content helps prevent constipation and the other digestive irregularities frequently seen with menstrual pain and cramps.

Fresh and dried fruits are excellent snack and dessert substitutes for cookies, candies, cakes, and other foods high in refined sugar. Though fruit is high in sugar, its high fiber content slows down absorption of the sugar into the blood circulation and helps stabilize the blood sugar level. I recommend, however, using fruit juices only in small quantities. Fruit juice does not contain the bulk or fiber of the whole fruit. As a result, it acts more like table sugar and can dramatically destabilize your blood sugar level when used in excess. In this case, less is better. If you want fruit juice on a more frequent basis, mix it half-and-half with water.

Seeds and Nuts. Seeds and nuts are the best sources of the two essential fatty acids, linoleic acid and linolenic acid.

These acids provide the raw materials your body needs to produce the muscle-relaxant prostaglandin hormones. Adequate levels of essential fatty acids in your diet are very important in treating and preventing endometriosis-related muscle cramps and inflammation. The best sources of both fatty acids are raw flax and pumpkin seeds. Sesame and sunflower seeds are excellent sources of linoleic acid alone. Seeds and nuts are excellent sources of the B-complex vitamins and vitamin E, important anti-stress factors for women with cramps; these nutrients also help to regulate hormonal balance. Seeds and nuts are also very high in other essential nutrients that women need, such as magnesium, calcium, and potassium. Particularly good to eat are sesame seeds, sunflower seeds, pistachios, pecans, and almonds. Because they are very high in calories, seeds and nuts should be eaten in small amounts.

The oils in seeds and nuts are very perishable, so avoid exposure to light, heat, and oxygen. Seeds and nuts should be eaten raw and unsalted to get the benefit of their essential fatty acids (which are good for your skin and hair) as well as to avoid the negative effects of too much salt. Shell them yourself, when possible. If you buy them already shelled, refrigerate them so their oils don't become rancid. They are a wonderful garnish on salads, vegetable dishes, and casseroles. They can also be eaten as a main source of protein in snacks and light meals.

Meat, Poultry, and Fish. I generally recommend eating meat only in small quantities or avoiding it altogether if you have fibroid and endometriosis symptoms. Beef, pork, lamb, and poultry contain saturated fats that produce the muscle-contracting F_2 Alpha prostaglandins. These hormones trigger muscle contraction and constriction in blood vessels, as well as inflammation, thereby worsening endometriosis-related cramps and the spread of endometrial implants.

If you do eat meat, I recommend emphasizing fish. Fish, unlike other meat, contains linolenic acid, one of the fatty acids that help to relax muscles through the beneficial prostaglandin pathway—specifically, the series-one and series-three prostaglandins. Fish are also excellent sources of minerals, especially iodine and potassium. Particularly good types of fish for women with menstrual cramps are salmon, tuna, mackerel, and trout.

If you include meat in your fibroid- and endometriosis-relief program, I recommend using it in very small amounts (3 ounces or less per day). Most Americans eat much more protein than is healthy. Excessive amounts of protein are difficult to digest and stress the kidneys. Except for fish, meat is also a main source of unhealthy saturated fats, which put you at higher risk of heart disease and cancer. Instead of using meat as your only source of protein, I recommend that you increase your intake of grains, beans, raw seeds, and nuts, which contain protein as well as many other important nutrients. For many years I have recommended that my patients use meat more as a garnish and a flavoring for casseroles, stir-fries, and soups. I also recommend buying the meat of organic, range-fed animals; this reduces the exposure to pesticides, antibiotics, and hormones. If you find meat difficult to digest, you may be deficient in hydrochloric acid. Try taking a small amount of hydrochloric acid with every meat-containing meal to see if your digestion improves.

Oils. You can use vegetable oils in small amounts for cooking, stir-frying, and sautéing. When you do, select an oil like corn oil that contains vitamin E. Vitamin E is an important nutrient in reducing the mood symptoms, fatigue, and cramps that occur at the onset of menstruation for women whose fibroids or endometriosis coexists with PMS. Vitamin E may help regulate hormone levels. This is important because high levels of estrogen stimulate the growth of fibroids and endometriosis. Women with these problems should use vitamin E in supplemental form (refer to Chapter 6 for more information). Other good oils for cooking are olive oil and canola oil.

Flax oil, which is notable for its beautiful golden color and delicious nutty flavor, can be used to enhance the flavor of rice, steamed vegetables, toast, popcorn, and many other foods. Many of my patients use it as a butter substitute. However, you cannot cook with flax oil because it is very perishable, sensitive to heat, light, and oxygen. Instead, you must first cook the food, then add the flax oil just before serving. Keep flax oil tightly capped and refrigerated. All oils should be cold-pressed to help ensure freshness and purity. Keep your oils refrigerated to avoid rancidity.

Foods to Avoid with Fibroids and Endometriosis

If you have fibroids or endometriosis, you should avoid or use only limited amounts of the foods described in this section. You will also notice that some of these foods are recognized as being high-stress or unhealthy foods for the body in general.

Dairy Products. Dairy products such as cheese, yogurt, milk, and cottage cheese should be avoided by women with fibroids or endometriosis. Because dairy products have traditionally been touted as one of the four basic food groups, this information may be a surprise. Dairy products are the main dietary source of arachidonic acid, the fat used by your body to produce muscle-contracting F_2 Alpha prostaglandins. These prostaglandins can increase pelvic pain, cramps, and inflammation characteristic of endometriosis. By deleting all dairy products from the diet, the severity of menstrual pain and cramps can be decreased by as much as one-third to one-half within one to two menstrual cycles.

The high saturated-fat content of many dairy products is a risk factor for excess estrogen levels in the body. Research studies have shown that vegetarian women eating a low fat, high fiber diet excrete two to three times more estrogen in their bowel movements and have 50 percent lower blood levels of estrogen than women eating a diet high in dairy and animal fats. Bacteria in the colon actually convert metabolites of cholesterol to forms of estrogen that can be reabsorbed from the digestive tract back into the body. This elevates the body's estrogen levels which is a trigger for fibroids and endometriosis and accelerates the spread of the disease. High estrogen levels have also been linked to heavy menstrual bleeding, another common complaint of women with these problems.

Dairy products have many other unhealthy effects on a woman's body. Many people are allergic to dairy products or lack the enzymes to digest milk. The result can be digestive problems such as bloating, gas, and bowel changes, which intensify with menstruation. This intolerance to dairy products can hamper the absorption and assimilation of calcium.

Because dairy products are a risk factor for fibroids and endometriosis, women who have depended on dairy products for their calcium intake naturally wonder about alternative sources. The many other good dietary sources of this essential nutrient include beans, peas, soybeans, sesame seeds, soup stock made from chicken or fish bones, and green leafy vegetables. For food preparation, soy milk, potato milk, and nut milk are excellent substitutes. You can also use a supplement containing calcium, magnesium, and vitamin D to make sure your intake is sufficient. Nondairy milks are available at health food stores and some supermarkets.

Fats. Saturated fats in general come from animal sources, and from a few vegetable sources such as palm oil or coconut oil. Like dairy products, they contain arachidonic acid, and therefore can intensify menstrual cramps by stimulating production of the muscle-contracting prostaglandins. Unfortunately, in the typical American diet, 40 percent of the calories come from fat. Most of this fat comes from unhealthy saturated sources such as dairy products, red meat, and eggs. This diet promotes heavy menstrual bleeding and even fibroid tumor growth in susceptible women. Excessive saturated fat intake is stressful to the liver, so the liver is less able to break down estrogen efficiently, leading to excess estrogen levels. Fibroids can worsen cramps when they grow to be too large, cutting off their own blood supply and pressing on the bladder and intestines.

Saturated fat, primarily from animal sources, also puts women at high risk of heart disease and cancers of the breast, uterus, and ovaries. Women on a high-fat diet also tend to accumulate excess weight more easily. Instead of foods high in saturated fats, eat more fruits, vegetables, grains, fish, and poultry. As often as possible, eat fresh and homemade foods prepared with a minimum of fats and oils. If you must eat packaged and processed foods, read the labels. Avoid those with a high fat content. Red meat should be used only in small amounts. Avoid or adapt recipes that call for large amounts of butter, cream, cheese, or other high-fat ingredients. Instead, flavor foods with garlic, onions, herbs, lemon juice, or a little olive oil (a monosaturated fat that doesn't increase your cholesterol level). Eat raw seeds and nuts rather than cooked ones (cooking alters the nature of the oils), and use them sparingly because of their high fat content.

Salt. Excessive salt intake can worsen the menstrual symptoms that frequently occur in women with fibroids and endometriosis. Too much dietary salt can increase bloating and fluid retention, particularly in women who have coexisting PMS. Too much salt intake can also increase high blood pressure and is a risk factor in the development of osteoporosis in menopausal women. Unfortunately, most processed food contains large amounts of salt. Frozen and canned foods are often loaded with salt. In fact, one frozen-food entree can contribute as much as one-half teaspoon of salt to your daily intake. Large amounts of salt are also commonly found in the American diet as table salt (sodium chloride), MSG (monosodium glutamate), and a variety of food additives. Fast foods such as hamburgers, hot dogs, french fries, pizza, and tacos are loaded with salt and saturated fats. Common foods such as soups, potato chips, cheese, olives, salad dressings, and catsup (to name only a few) are also very high in salt. To make matters worse, many people add too much salt while cooking and seasoning their meals.

Women with fibroids and endometriosis should avoid adding salt to their meals. For flavor, use seasonings like garlic, herbs, spices, and lemon juice. Avoid processed foods that are high in salt, such as canned foods, olives, pickles, potato chips, tortilla chips, catsup, and salad dressings. Learn to read labels and look for the word sodium (salt). If it appears high on the list of ingredients, don't buy the product. Many items in health food stores are labeled "no salt added." Some supermarkets also offer "no added salt" foods in their diet or health food sections.

Alcohol. Women with fibroids or endometriosis should avoid alcohol entirely or consume it only in small amounts. Like dairy products and saturated fats, alcohol is stressful to the liver and can affect the liver's ability to metabolize hormones efficiently. Excessive alcohol intake has been associated with both lack of ovulation and elevated estrogen levels, which can trigger the growth and spread of endometrial implants in susceptible women, worsening menstrual cramps and pain. It can also trigger heavy bleeding in estrogen-sensitive women with fibroids and endometriosis. Excessive estrogen can worsen the congestive symptoms of menstrual pain and cramps. Estrogen causes fluid and salt retention in the body. When levels are too high, the body can retain excessive amounts of fluid during the premenstrual and menstrual phases of the month.

Alcohol also depletes the body's B-complex vitamins and minerals such as magnesium by disrupting carbohydrate metabolism. Because minerals are important in regulating muscle tension, an alcohol-based nutritional deficiency can worsen muscle spasms at the time of menstruation. Depletion of magnesium and vitamin B complex can also intensify menstrual fatigue and mood swings.

Though alcohol has a relaxing effect and can enhance the taste of food, I recommend that women with fibroids or endometriosis avoid or limit its use, particularly in the early stages of treatment. This is even more important for women who have coexisting PMS. For these women, the use of alcohol can aggravate the PMS-related mood swings, irritability, and other symptoms.

If you entertain a great deal and enjoy social drinking, try using nonalcoholic beverages. A nonalcoholic cocktail such as mineral water with a twist of lime or lemon or a dash of bitters is a good substitute. "Near beer" is a nonalcoholic beer substitute that tastes quite good. Light wine and beer—in small amounts—have a lower alcohol content than hard liquor, liqueurs, and regular wine.

Sugar. Like alcohol, sugar depletes the body's B-complex vitamins and minerals, which can worsen muscle tension and irritability as well as nervous tension and anxiety. Lack of certain B vitamins also hampers the liver's ability to handle fats, including the fat-based hormone estrogen. One particular B vitamin, B_6, is also needed for the production of beneficial types of prostaglandins that have relaxant and anti-inflammatory effects, both important for the treatment of endometriosis.

Unfortunately, sugar addiction is very common in our society in people of all ages. Many people use sweet foods as a way to deal with their frustrations and other upsets. As a result, most Americans eat too much sugar—the average American eats 120 pounds each year. Many convenience foods, such as salad dressing, catsup, and relish, contain high levels of both sugar and salt. Sugar is the main ingredient in soft drinks and in desserts such as candies, cookies, cakes, and ice cream. Highly sugared foods also lead to tooth loss through tooth decay and gum disease. Of even greater significance is the fact that excessive sugar intake can aggravate diabetes and blood sugar imbalances.

Try to satisfy your sweet tooth instead with healthier foods, such as fruit or grain-based desserts like oatmeal cookies made with fruit or honey. You will find that small amounts of these foods can satisfy your cravings. Instead of disrupting your mood and energy level, they actually have a healthful and balancing effect.

Caffeine. Coffee, black tea, soft drinks, and chocolate—all these foods contain caffeine, a stimulant that many women use to increase their energy level and alertness and decrease fatigue. Caffeine is even used in many over-the-counter menstrual remedies that women with early-stage endometriosis often take for symptom relief. Unfortunately, caffeine has many negative effects on the body. For example, caffeine used in excess increases anxiety, irritability, and mood swings. This can be a real problem for women in whom PMS coexists with fibroids or endometriosis. Caffeine also depletes the body's stores of B-complex vitamins and essential minerals, so long-term use can increase fibroid- and endometriosis-related pain, cramps, and bleeding by disrupting both carbohydrate metabolism and healthy liver function. Many menopausal women also complain that caffeine increases the number of hot flashes. Coffee, black tea, chocolate, and caffeinated soft drinks all act to inhibit iron absorption, thus worsening anemia.

How to Substitute Healthy Ingredients in Recipes

Learning how to make substitutions for high-stress ingredients in recipes allows you to use your favorite recipes without compromising your health and well-being. Many recipes include ingredients that women with cramps need to avoid, like dairy products, salt, sugar, chocolate, and wheat. By eliminating the high-stress foods and replacing them with healthier ingredients, you can still make almost any recipe that you choose. I have recommended this technique for years to my patients, who have found with delight that they can still make their favorite dishes, but in much healthier versions.

Some women choose to totally eliminate the high-stress ingredients from a recipe. For example, you might make a pasta and tomato sauce, but eliminate the Parmesan cheese topping, or make a Greek salad without the feta cheese. Some of my patients even make pizza without cheese, layering tomato sauce and lots of vegetables on top of a pizza crust. In many cases, the high-stress ingredients are not necessary in order to make foods taste good; always remember, they can worsen your symptoms.

If you want to retain a particular high-stress ingredient, you can substantially reduce the amount you use, while still retaining the flavor and taste. Most of us have palates jaded by too much salt, fat, sugar, and other flavorings. In many dishes, we taste only the additives and never really enjoy the delicious flavor of the foods themselves. During the years that I have substituted low-stress ingredients in my cooking, I have come to enjoy the subtle taste of the dishes much more. Also, I find that my health and vitality continue to improve with the deletion of high-stress ingredients from my food. The following information tells how to substitute healthy ingredients in your own recipes. The substitutions are simple to make and should benefit your health greatly.

How to Substitute for Dairy Products

Decrease the amount of cow's milk cheese you use in food preparation and cooking. If you must use cow's milk cheese, decrease the amount by one-half to two-thirds so that it becomes a flavoring or garnish rather than a major source of fat and protein. You can often replace cheese in recipes with soft tofu. I have done this with lasagna, layering the lasagna noodles with tofu and tomato sauce and topping with melted soy cheese for a delicious dish. The tofu, which is bland, takes on the taste of the tomato sauce. If you cannot give up cow's milk products, try to use the lower-fat cheeses now available. Goat's or sheep's milk cheese in small amounts can also replace cow's milk cheese, because the fat they contain is more easily emulsified in the body.

Use soy cheese in food preparation and cooking. Soy cheese is an excellent substitute for cow's milk cheese. It is lower in fat and salt, and the fat that it contains isn't saturated. Health food stores offer many brands in many different flavors, such as mozzarella, cheddar, American, and jack. The quality of these products keeps improving all the time. You can use soy cheese as a perfect cheese substitute in sandwiches, salads, pizzas, lasagnas, and casseroles.

Replace milk in recipes. For cow's milk, substitute potato milk, soy milk, nut milk, or grain milk. Soy milk and nut milk are available at most health food stores. Soy milk is particularly good and comes in many flavors; it can be found in some supermarkets. Many nondairy milks are good sources of calcium and can be used for drinking, eating, or baking. One of my personal favorites is a nondairy milk made from an all-vegetable potato base. It is creamy and sweet and tastes very similar to the best cow's milk, with none of the unhealthy characteristics of dairy products. Even my 10-year-old daughter likes it. The potato-based milk is high in calcium and can be bought dry so that you can store it. It mixes easily in water and can be used exactly as you use cow's milk for beverages, cooking, and baking. The potato milk is available through *The LifeCycles Center.*

Substitute flax oil for butter. Flax oil is the best substitute for butter that I've found. It is a golden, rich oil that looks and tastes quite a bit like butter. It is delicious on anything you'd normally top with butter—toast, rice, popcorn, steamed vegetables, potatoes. Flax oil is extremely high in essential fatty acids— the type of fat that is very healthy for a woman's body. Essential fatty acids help promote normal hormonal function. Flax oil is quite perishable because it is sensitive to heat and light, so keep it refrigerated. You can't cook with it—always cook the food first and then add the flax oil before serving. There are so many health benefits to flax oil that I recommend it highly. You can find it in health food stores or order it from *The LifeCycles Center.*

How to Substitute for Caffeinated Foods and Beverages

Drink substitutes for coffee and black tea. The best substitutes are the grain-based coffee beverages like Pero, Postum, and Cafix. Some women find it difficult to discontinue coffee abruptly, because they suffer withdrawal symptoms such as headaches. If this is a concern for you, decrease your total coffee intake gradually to one-half to one cup per day. Use coffee substitutes for your other cups. This will help prevent withdrawal symptoms.

Use decaffeinated coffee or tea as a transition beverage. If you cannot give up coffee, you can start by substituting water-process decaffeinated coffee for the real thing. Then try to wean yourself from coffee altogether.

Use herbal teas for energy and vitality. Many women drink coffee for the pick-up they get from it. Those morning cups of coffee allow them to wake up and function through the day. Use ginger instead. It is a great herbal stimulant that won't wreck your health. To make ginger tea, grate a few teaspoons of fresh ginger root into a pot of hot water. Boil and steep. Serve with honey.

Substitute carob for chocolate. Unsweetened carob tastes like chocolate but is far more nutritious. It is a member of the legume family and is high in calcium. You can purchase it in chunk form as a substitute for chocolate candy, or in a powder for baking or drinks. Be careful, however, not to over-indulge; carob, like chocolate, is high in calories and fat. It should be considered a treat and a cooking aid to be used only in small amounts.

How to Substitute for Sugar

Cut the amount of sweetener in your recipes by one-third to one-half. This can be done easily without changing the taste of most dishes. Americans tend to be addicted to sugar. Most of us grew up on highly sugared soft drinks, candy, and rich pastries—no wonder the incidence of diabetes is soaring among our population. I have found that as women decrease their sugar intake, most begin to really enjoy the subtle flavors of the foods they eat.

Substitute concentrated sweeteners. Concentrated sweeteners such as honey and maple syrup have a sweeter taste per quantity used than table sugar. Using these substitutes will enable you to cut down on the amount of sugar used. If you use a concentrated sweetener in place of sugar in an ordinary recipe, reduce the liquid content in the recipe by one-fourth cup. If no liquid is used in the recipe, add 3 to 5 tablespoons of flour for each three-fourths cup of concentrated sweetener.

Substitute fruit for sugar in pastries. In making muffins and cookies, you may want to try deleting sugar altogether and adding extra fruits and nuts.

How to Substitute for Salt

Substitute potassium-based products for table salt (sodium chloride). Potassium-based products, such as Morton's Salt Substitute, are much healthier and will not aggravate heart disease or hypertension.

Substitute powdered seaweeds like kelp or nori to season vegetables, grains, and salads. They are high in essential iodine and trace elements.

Use herbs instead of salt for flavoring. Their flavors are much more subtle and will help even the most jaded palates appreciate the taste of vegetables and meats.

Use low-sodium-content liquid flavoring agents. Low-salt soy sauce and Bragg's Amino Acids, a liquid soybean-based flavoring agent, are delicious when used as salt substitutes in cooking. When added to soups, casseroles, stir-fries, and other dishes at the end of the cooking process, a small amount provides intense flavoring.

How to Substitute for Wheat Flour

Use whole grain nonwheat flour. Substitute whole grain nonwheat flours, such as rice or barley flour. These whole grain flours are much higher in essential nutrients, including vitamin B complex and many minerals. They are also higher in fiber content. Rice flour makes excellent cookies, cakes, and other pastries. For pie crusts, barley flour is better.

How to Substitute for Alcohol

Use low-alcohol or nonalcoholic products for cooking. Substitute low-alcohol or nonalcoholic wine or beer when cooking or preparing sauces and marinades. You will retain much of the flavor that alcohol imparts and you'll decrease the stress factor substantially.

Substitutes for Common High-Stress Ingredients

3/4 cup sugar	1/2 cup honey
	1/4 cup molasses
	1/2 cup maple syrup
	1/2 oz. barley malt
	1 cup apple butter
	2 cups apple juice
1 cup milk	1 cup soy, potato, nut, or grain milk
1 tablespoon butter	1 tablespoon flax oil (must be used raw and unheated)
1/2 teaspoon salt	1 tablespoon miso
	1/2 teaspoon potassium chloride salt substitute
	1/2 teaspoon Mrs. Dash, Spike
	1/2 teaspoon herbs (basil, tarragon, oregano, etc.)
1-1/2 cups cocoa	1 cup powdered carob
1 square chocolate	3/4 tablespoon powdered carob
1 tablespoon coffee	1 tablespoon decaffeinated coffee
	1 tablespoon Pero, Postum, Cafix, or other grain-based coffee substitute
4 ounces wine	4 ounces light wine
8 ounces beer	8 ounces near beer
1 cup wheat flour	1 cup barley flour (pie crust)
	1 cup rice flour (cookies, cakes, breads)

5

Menus,
Meal Plans, &
Recipes

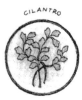

CILANTRO

$\mathcal{T}$his chapter addresses the pleasant subjects of meal planning and dining. While women with fibroids or endometriosis need to give up high-stress foods to gain symptom relief, a therapeutic diet can be delicious and pleasurable to the senses. As you make the transition to better dietary habits, not only are the foods enjoyable to eat, but you will gain the tremendous benefit of improved health and well-being.

I began to work with meal planning many years ago when I was attempting to treat my own health problems. My work in nutrition goes back almost 20 years, when I first saw the dramatic benefits that a low-stress, high-nutrient diet had on my menstrual cramps and PMS symptoms. My health problems cleared up beautifully when I made the necessary nutritional changes. I am healthier now in my late forties than I was as a teenager or in my twenties, because I no longer have any of the problems that were bothering me then. I give a great deal of credit for my current excellent health to my continuing emphasis on good dietary habits.

Upon learning the importance of diet and nutrition, most of my patients have asked me for specific menus, meal plans, and recipes to help them implement their own self-care programs. Unfortunately, very few specific resources are available. No cookbooks adequately address a woman's needs for specific nutrients. Most contain recipes that are too high in the nutrients that can worsen cramps—animal fats, chocolate, sugar, and salt. More nutrition-conscious cookbooks present low-calorie "light dishes" that eliminate the high-stress ingredients, but still don't give women with fibroids or endometriosis the therapeutic levels of specific nutrients they need. As a result, I've had to develop these resources for women myself.

This chapter contains menus and recipes that I've given to patients, over the years, with very beneficial therapeutic results. Because many women lead busy lives and have many demands on their time, I've devised recipes that are quick and easy to prepare. I've found that anything too complicated doesn't work for either me or my patients. Best of all, these recipes are delicious as well as healthful. I hope that you find trying these new dishes to be a delightful adventure as well as a boon to your health.

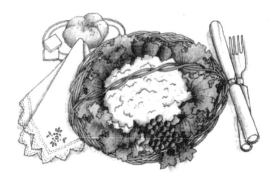

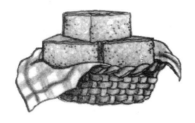

Breakfast Menus

These breakfast menus have been developed to reduce and prevent symptoms of fibroids and endometriosis. All the dishes contain high levels of the essential nutrients that women with these problems need; the recipes call for no high-stress ingredients.

Breakfast has been one of the easiest meals for my patients to restructure along healthier lines. You probably eat breakfast at home alone or with family members. It tends to be a smaller and simpler meal. You may want to make healthful dietary changes in your breakfast first and then move on to lunch and dinner. Starred (*) recipes can be found in this chapter.

*Flax shake
Rice cakes

* Oatmeal cereal #1
* Relaxant herb tea

*Instant flax cereal
*Pain relief tea

*Tofu cereal
Rose hip tea

*Millet cereal
*Nondairy milk breakfast
    shake

*Brown rice cereal
Spring water

*Corn muffins
*Rice pancakes
Banana
Vanilla nondairy milk

Raw sesame butter
Roasted grain beverage (coffee
    substitute)

Lunch and Dinner Menus

Here is a variety of menus you can choose from when planning your meals. These dishes contain many nutritious and healthful ingredients for fibroid and endometriosis relief. Use these menus as helpful guidelines throughout the entire month. Your nutritional status on a day-by-day basis determines in part how likely you are to have fibroid or endometriosis symptoms. These dishes should help to diminish the severity of your symptoms because they eliminate high-stress foods. Starred (*) recipes are included in this chapter.

Soup Meals	Salad Meals
*Split pea soup	*Spinach salad
*Corn muffins	*Corn muffins with flax oil
*Fresh applesauce	
	*Beet salad
Potato-kale soup	Rye bread with fresh fruit
*Cole slaw	preserves
Rye bread with flax oil	
Dried figs	Romaine salad
	Rye crackers
*Vegetable soup	Orange slices
*Steamed kale	
*Baked potato with flax oil	*Cole slaw
Apple slices	*Potato salad
	Melon
*Carrot soup	
*Broccoli with lemon	
Brown rice	
Banana	
Tomato soup	
*Potato salad	
Celery spears	

One-Dish Vegetable Meals

*Vegetarian tacos with
   low-salt salsa

*Tofu and almond stir-fry
Steamed rice

*Pasta with oil and garlic
Green salad

Hummus and tahini
Rye bread
Mixed raw vegetable
   slices

*Rice and almond tabouli
Black olives

Meat Meals

*Poached salmon
Brown rice
*Steamed carrots

*Broiled tuna
*Baked potato with flax oil
*Broccoli with lemon

Broiled trout with dill
Mixed green salad
*Green peas and onions

Grilled shrimp
*Wild rice
*Steamed kale

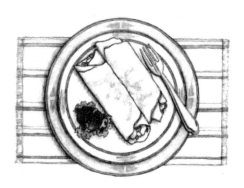

Breakfast Recipes

Beverages

These drinks are made with specific herbs, fruits, raw seeds, and nuts that are recommended for preventing and treating your symptoms. The ingredients contain high levels of essential nutrients that help regulate your hormonal balance and relax tension in the muscles of the pelvis and lower extremities. You can enjoy these drinks throughout the month, as their high mineral and other nutrient content is beneficial for the entire body.

Relaxant Herb Tea *Serves 2*

1 pint water
1 teaspoon chamomile
  leaves
1 teaspoon peppermint
  leaves
1 teaspoon honey
  (if desired)

Bring the water to a boil. Place herbs in water and stir. Turn heat to low and simmer for 15 minutes. *Peppermint and chamomile are both muscle relaxants and antispasmodic herbs, so they can provide relief of pain and cramping caused by fibroids and endometriosis. They also help calm the mood.*

Pain Relief Tea *Serves 2*

1 pint water
1 teaspoon grated fresh
  ginger root
1 teaspoon raspberry leaves
1 teaspoon honey
  (if desired)

Bring water to a boil. Place herbs in water and stir. Turn heat to low and simmer for 15 minutes. *Ginger has both pain-relieving (analgesic) and antinausea properties. Raspberry leaves have uterine relaxant properties and help relieve diarrhea. This is a helpful combination for relief of fibroid and endometriosis symptoms.*

Flax Shake *Serves 2*

4 tablespoons raw flax
    seeds
2 bananas
6 oz. water
6 oz. apple juice

Grind flax seeds to a powder using a coffee or seed grinder. Place powdered flax seeds in a blender. Add remaining ingredients and blend. *Because of the whole flax seed, this recipe is high in essential fatty acids, calcium, magnesium, and potassium, making it a very powerful recipe for treating fibroids and their symptoms.*

**Nondairy Milk
Breakfast Shake** *Serves 2*

2 cups nondairy milk
2 oz. soft tofu
3 tablespoons flax oil
1 large banana
3/4 cup berries (straw-
    berries, boysenberries,
    blueberries, or rasp-
    berries)

Combine all ingredients in a blender. Blend until smooth and serve. *This delicious, creamy shake is excellent for relief of fibroid- or endometriosis-related cramps and pain because it is high in essential fatty acids, calcium, vitamin C, and potassium.*

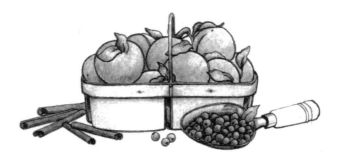

Cereals, Muffins, and Pancakes

Most American breakfasts include wheat and dairy products, such as yogurt, wheat toast, wheat cereal with milk, sweet rolls, and other wheat-based pastries. As I explained in Chapter 4, dairy products and wheat can worsen the symptoms of fibroids, endometriosis, and PMS (which often occurs concurrently). I have included in this section three types of simple, alternative dishes you can make to replace wheat and dairy products at breakfast. They are based on whole flax seed, soy, and gluten-free grains, all of which can be useful in reducing your symptoms. Gluten is the protein found in wheat that can trigger symptoms of bloating, digestive disturbances, and fatigue.

Instant Flax Cereal   *Serves 1*

4 tablespoons raw flax seeds
4 to 8 oz. vanilla-flavored nondairy milk
1/2 banana, sliced
sweetener (to taste)

Grind raw flax seeds into a powder using a seed or coffee grinder. Place powder in a cereal bowl and slowly add nondairy milk, stirring the mixture together. The flax mixture will thicken to a texture like cream of rice or oatmeal. Top the cereal with sliced bananas. Add sweetener if desired. Eat the mixture right away; flax seeds are sensitive to light, air, and temperature. This cereal should be eaten cold. Do not cook this cereal.

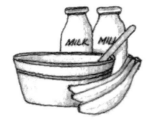

Tofu Cereal   *Serves 2*

4 oz. soft tofu
2 oz. vanilla-flavored
   nondairy milk
2 tablespoons flax oil
1 banana
1 apple
15 raw almonds
sweetener (if desired)

Combine all ingredients in a food processor. Blend until creamy. Pour into a bowl and serve. *This is a helpful cereal for fibroid- and endometriosis-related cramps because it is high in essential fatty acids, calcium, magnesium, and potassium.*

Millet Cereal   *Serves 2*

1 cup millet
2 cups water
1 teaspoon canola oil
4 oz. vanilla-flavored
   nondairy milk
1 tablespoon honey
1 tablespoon raw sun-
   flower seeds
1 tablespoon raw sesame
   seeds

Wash millet with cold water. Combine millet, water, and canola oil in a pot and bring to a boil. Turn heat to low; cover and cook without stirring about 25 to 35 minutes, until millet is soft. Don't check before 20 minutes, because too much steam will be lost. Fluff up the millet and spoon into serving bowls. Add the remaining ingredients. Mix and serve. *Raw sunflower and sesame seeds are excellent sources of essential fatty acids, calcium, magnesium, and potassium, which help to relieve pain and cramp symptoms.*

Brown Rice Cereal   *Serves 2*

1 cup brown rice

2 cups water

1 pinch sea salt

10 raw almonds, chopped

1 teaspoon honey

2 oz. vanilla-flavored
   nondairy milk or apple
   juice (if desired)

3 tablespoons flax oil

Wash rice in cold water.
Combine rice, water, and salt in a
pot and bring to a boil. Stir and
turn heat to low. Cover the pot
and cook 25 to 35 minutes. Don't
open the pot and check before 20
minutes, because too much steam
will be lost. Add the remaining
ingredients. Mix and serve.

Oatmeal Cereal #1   *Serves 2*

1-1/2 cups water

2/3 cup oats

2 tablespoons raw flax
   seeds, ground

2 to 4 oz. vanilla-flavored
   nondairy milk

1/2 banana

2 teaspoons honey

Boil water in a pot. Stir in oats
and return to a boil. Reduce heat
to medium low. Cook uncovered
for 5 minutes, stirring occasionally. Remove from heat; let stand
a few minutes. Stir in ground raw
flax seeds; add nondairy milk,
sliced banana, and honey. Serve.

Oatmeal Cereal #2   *Serves 2*

1-1/2 cups water

2/3 cup oats

3 tablespoons flax oil

2 teaspoons maple syrup

Boil water in a pot; stir in oats.
Return mixture to a boil; reduce
heat to medium low. Cook
uncovered for 5 minutes, stirring
occasionally. Remove from heat;
let stand for a few minutes. Stir
in flax oil and maple syrup.
Serve.

Brown Rice Pancakes   *Serves 4*

1 cup rice flour
1/4 teaspoon salt
2 cups cooked brown rice
1 cup vanilla-flavored
   nondairy milk
1 egg, separated
4 tablespoons flax oil
4 teaspoons maple syrup

Combine rice flour and salt in a large bowl; add rice. Beat nondairy milk and egg yolk together, then add to dry mixture. Beat egg white until stiff. Fold egg white into batter. Pour batter onto a lightly oiled hot griddle or frying pan. Cook on medium heat. Turn pancakes when they begin to brown. Top with flax oil and maple syrup and serve.

Wild Rice Pancakes   *Serves 4*

1 cup rice flour
1/4 teaspoon salt
2 cups cooked wild rice
1 cup vanilla-flavored
   nondairy milk
1 egg, separated
4 tablespoons flax oil
6 tablespoons strawberry or
   raspberry fruit puree or
   jam (no added sugar)

Combine rice flour and salt in a large bowl; add wild rice. Beat nondairy milk and egg yolk together and add to dry mixture. Beat egg white until stiff. Fold egg white into batter. Pour batter onto a lightly oiled hot griddle or frying pan. Cook on medium heat. Turn pancakes when they begin to get crisp and brown. Top with flax oil and fruit puree or jam. Serve.

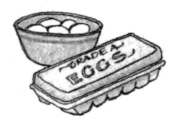

Corn Muffins
Serves 8 to 10

2 tablespoons canola oil
3 tablespoons honey
2 eggs, beaten
2 cups vanilla-flavored
    nondairy milk
2 cups cornmeal
1/2 cup rice flour
1/2 teaspoon salt
1 teaspoon baking powder
1/2 teaspoon baking soda

Combine oil, honey, eggs, and nondairy milk in a bowl; mix well and set aside. Mix together cornmeal, rice flour, salt, baking powder, and baking soda. Combine wet and dry ingredients and mix until batter is smooth. Spoon batter into well-oiled muffin tins and bake about 20 minutes at 425° F. *Muffins are delicious with fresh flax oil or blackberry preserves and raw almond butter.*

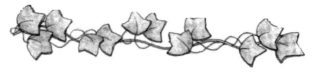

Spreads and Sauces

These spreads and sauces contain highly concentrated levels of ingredients that help to relax fibroid- and endometriosis-related pain and muscle tension and help to relieve congestion. Serve with rice cakes, crackers, corn bread, or even spread on a banana for a delicious treat.

Flax Spread
Serves 2

6 tablespoons raw flax seeds
juice of 1/2 lemon
1/2 teaspoon Bragg's
    Liquid Amino Acids
2 tablespoons water

Grind flax seeds to a powder using a coffee or seed grinder. Place powder in a small bowl and add the remaining ingredients. Mix into a paste. Use as a spread with rice cakes or crackers.

Fresh Applesauce   *Serves 2*

2-1/2 apples
1/2 cup fresh apple juice
1/2 teaspoon cinnamon
1/2 teaspoon ginger

Peel apples and cut into quarters; remove cores. Combine all ingredients in a food processor. Blend until smooth.

**Sesame-Tofu
Spread**   *Makes 1-1/2 cups*

1/4 cup soft tofu
3/8 cup raw sesame butter
1/4 cup honey

Combine all ingredients in a blender. Serve with rice cakes or crackers.

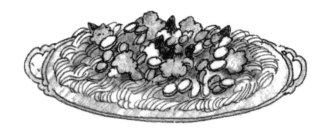

Lunch and Dinner Recipes

These high-nutrient, healthful lunch and dinner dishes are designed to help prevent and relieve your symptoms. The ingredients in the recipes do not include red meat, dairy products, poultry, or wheat, all of which can worsen your symptoms. Mix and match these dishes as you please. You might combine soups and salads or starches and vegetables for a complete meal. The main course dishes are all extremely healthful for women with fibroids or endometriosis. You can enjoy these dishes particularly during the second half of your menstrual cycle when your symptoms are worse, but for optimal health and well-being, I recommend their use all month long.

Soups

4 tomatoes, diced
1 onion, chopped
1 turnip, chopped
1/2 leek, chopped
1 cup green peas
2 carrots, chopped
8 mushrooms, sliced
1 bay leaf
1/2 tablespoon thyme
1/2 tablespoon oregano
1/2 teaspoon sea salt or
    salt substitute
1 to 1-1/2 quarts water
1/4 bunch parsley,
    chopped

Vegetable Soup   *Serves 6*

Place all ingredients in a pot. Cover with the water. Bring to a boil, then turn heat to low. Cook for 45 minutes. Pour the soup into individual serving dishes. Garnish with chopped parsley.

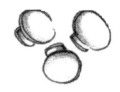

1 cup dried split peas
1/2 onion, chopped
1 small carrot, sliced
1 quart water
1/4 to 1/2 teaspoon sea
    salt or salt substitute

Split Pea Soup   *Serves 4*

Wash peas. Place peas, onion, and carrot in a pot. Add the water. Bring to a boil, then turn heat to low and cover pot. Cook for 45 minutes. Add sea salt and continue to cook until peas are soft.

Soup may be cooled and then pureed in a blender if you prefer a creamy texture.

Lentil Soup *Serves 4*

1 cup dried lentils
1/2 onion, chopped
1/2 cup chopped carrots
1 to 1-1/2 quarts water
1 teaspoon brown rice miso

Wash lentils. Place all ingredients in a pot. Bring to a boil, then turn heat to low. Cover pot and simmer until lentils are soft. Vary the amount of water depending on the desired thickness of the soup.

Carrot Soup *Serves 4*

4 cups peeled and sliced
  carrots
1-1/4 cups diced onions
1/2 cup chopped sweet
  red pepper
4 cups vegetable broth
1-1/2 tablespoons grated
  ginger root
1-1/2 cup vanilla-flavored
  nondairy milk

Combine carrots, onions, red pepper, vegetable broth, and ginger in a large pot; cook for 30 minutes or until carrots are tender. Strain vegetables and reserve broth. Puree vegetables in a food processor. Blend together and puree broth, nondairy milk, and vegetables. Return soup to cooking pot. Cook on low for 5 minutes. Serve.

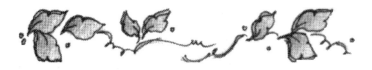

Salads

Romaine Salad *Serves 4*

1 head romaine lettuce
1/4 red onion, chopped
4 mushrooms, sliced

Combine all ingredients in a large salad bowl. Serve with an olive oil or flax oil and vinegar dressing. *Avoid cheese or cream dressings.*

3 medium steamed beets, diced
1 medium red onion, chopped
1/2 bunch parsley, chopped
1/2 red pepper, diced
1/4 cup sunflower seeds

Beet Salad
Serves 4

Combine all ingredients in a large salad bowl. Serve with an oil-and-vinegar dressing. *Avoid cheese or cream-based dressing. This salad is great in summer.*

8 medium red potatoes
1 cup chopped celery
1/2 cup finely chopped parsley
1/2 cup chopped sweet, raw onions
1/2 cup chopped green pepper

Potato Salad
Serves 6

Steam potatoes for approximately 45 minutes. Cool and cube. Combine celery, parsley, pepper, and onions with potatoes; mix thoroughly. Add a small amount of your favorite dressing. *Both vinaigrette and low-calorie mayonnaise are delicious on potato salad.*

1/2 teaspoon celery seeds
1/2 teaspoon poppy seeds
1/2 teaspoon dill seeds
2 cups finely shredded red cabbage
1-1/2 cups finely shredded green cabbage

Cole Slaw
Serves 4

Crush or grind seeds and add to shredded cabbage. Serve with favorite dressing (oil-and-vinegar or honey dressing preferred). *The herbs used are high in calcium and magnesium as well as iron.*

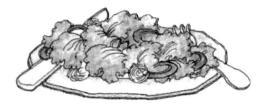

Spinach Salad *Serves 4*

1 bunch spinach, chopped
1/2 small red onion,
   chopped
1/3 cup diced red pepper
1/2 cup mung bean sprouts
2 oz. firm tofu, diced
1/4 cup raw sunflower seeds

Combine all ingredients in a large salad bowl. Serve with your favorite nondairy dressing.

Grains and Starches

Wild Rice *Serves 4*

2/3 cup wild rice
2-1/2 cups cold water
1/2 teaspoon sea salt

Wash rice with cold water. Combine all ingredients in a cooking pot and bring to a rapid boil. Turn flame to low, cover, and cook without stirring (about 45 minutes) until rice is tender but not mushy. Uncover and fluff with a fork. Cook an additional 5 minutes, then serve.

Kasha *Serves 4*

1 cup kasha (buckwheat
   groats)
3-1/4 cups water
pinch salt

Bring ingredients to a boil, lower heat, and simmer for 25 minutes or until soft. The grains should be fluffy, like rice. *For breakfast, blend in blender with water until creamy. Add almond milk, sesame milk, or sunflower milk, and cinnamon, apple butter, ginger, raisins, or berries.*

Baked Sweet Potato   *Serves 4*

4 sweet potatoes
1 tablespoon canola oil
1 tablespoon flax oil for
each potato

Preheat oven to 400° F. Wash the potatoes, then rub with canola oil. Bake for 45 to 60 minutes, or until soft when pierced with a fork. Garnish with flax oil. Honey, maple syrup, or chopped raw pecans may also be used.

Baked Potato   *Serves 4*

4 russet or Idaho potatoes
1 tablespoon vegetable oil
1 tablespoon flax oil for
each potato

Preheat oven to 400° F. Wash the potatoes, rub them with vegetable oil, and bake for 45 to 60 minutes, or until soft when pierced with a fork. Garnish with flax oil. Other garnishes can include chopped green onions, soy cheese, and low-salt salsa.

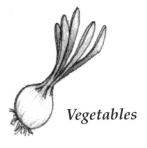

Vegetables

Steamed Kale   *Serves 4*

1 bunch kale (stems
removed), chopped
juice of 1 lemon
2 to 3 tablespoons olive oil
pinch of sea salt

Steam the kale until tender. Dress with lemon juice, olive oil, and sea salt. *Kale is an excellent vegetable for women with menstrual pain and cramps, and I recommend its frequent use. Swiss chard and mustard greens, two other excellent vegetables for women with menstrual discomfort, can be prepared and dressed the same way.*

Steamed Cabbage
Serves 4

1 small head cabbage,
   quartered
1 teaspoon chopped parsley
1 teaspoon olive oil

Steam cabbage until tender. Sprinkle with olive oil and parsley.

Broccoli with Lemon
Serves 4

1 pound broccoli
juice of 1/2 lemon
4 tablespoons flax oil

Cut the broccoli into small flowerets; steam for 6 minutes or until tender. Squeeze lemon juice over broccoli and add the flax oil. Mix and serve. *For an different taste treat, try substituting Bragg's Liquid Amino Acids for the lemon juice.*

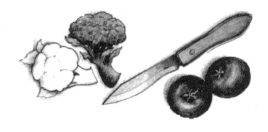

Cauliflower with Flax Oil
Serves 4

1 medium head cauliflower
4 tablespoons flax oil
1 teaspoon salt substitute

Break the cauliflower into small flowerets. Steam 10 minutes or until tender. Toss with flax oil and salt substitute.

Steamed Carrots
Serves 4

8 medium carrots, sliced
1 tablespoon maple syrup

Steam carrots until soft. Top with maple syrup.

Whipped
Acorn Squash   *Serves 4*

2 acorn squash
2 to 3 oz. apple juice
pinch ground cinnamon

Peel the acorn squash and cut into large pieces. Steam the squash until tender. Place in a food processor with the remaining ingredients, blending to a smooth consistency.

Green Beans
and Almonds   *Serves 4*

1 pound green beans
2 oz. raw almonds, chopped
2 tablespoons flax oil
1/4 teaspoon salt substitute

Steam green beans until tender. Toss with the almond bits, flax oil, and sea salt for a buttery flavor. If you don't care for the taste of flax oil, substitute a vinaigrette.

Green Peas and Onions   *Serves 4*

1 cup green peas
1/2 cup diced onions

Heat water to boiling, then turn heat to low. Add peas and onions and simmer for 20 minutes or until peas are tender.

Zucchini and Eggplant   *Serves 4*

2 medium zucchini, diced
1 cup cubed eggplant
1 small onion, chopped
1 clove garlic, minced
1/2 teaspoon basil
1 teaspoon oregano
1 tablespoon olive oil
1/8 teaspoon salt

Sauté zucchini, eggplant, and onion in a frying pan with a small amount of water. Add the remaining ingredients. Cook until tender, stirring constantly.

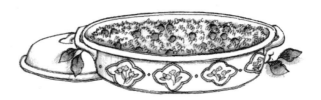

Main Dishes

Rice and Almond Tabouli *Serves 6*

2 cups cooked brown rice
1 cup chopped parsley
1/2 cup chopped fresh mint
1/2 medium red onion, diced
1 medium tomato, diced
1 oz. almonds, chopped
juice of 1 lemon
2 tablespoons olive oil
1 teaspoon cumin
1 teaspoon oregano
1/4 teaspoon salt

Place rice in a bowl. Mix in parsley, mint, red onion, tomato, and chopped almonds. Combine these ingredients well. Add lemon juice and olive oil; mix. Add cumin, oregano, and salt to the salad and mix well. *This is the ultimate delicious and healthy tabouli recipe. It is great served with hummus and tahini (see following recipe).*

Hummus and Tahini *Serves 4*

3/4 cup raw unhulled
    sesame seeds
1-3/4 cup cooked garbanzo
    beans
1 cup water or cooking
    liquid from beans
1 clove raw garlic
juice of 1 lemon
2 tablespoons olive oil
1/4 teaspoon salt

Grind sesame seeds into a powder using a seed or coffee grinder. (Raw sesame butter, available from most health food stores, may be substituted.) Combine ground sesame seeds, garbanzo beans, water, garlic, lemon juice, olive oil, and salt in a food processor. Blend to the consistency of a smooth dip. Serve as a dip with pita bread, rye bread, and fresh vegetables. *This is great served with rice tabouli (see previous recipe).*

6 oz. cooked black beans
6 oz. cooked lentils or
    great northern beans
1/4 red pepper, diced
1/4 small red onion, diced
2 oz. diced celery
1 cup cooked brown rice
6 leaves romaine lettuce
2 tablespoons chopped
    green onions

Two-Bean Dish   *Serves 2*

In two separate bowls, combine each bean portion with half of the red pepper, red onion, and celery. Mix well. Arrange leaves of romaine lettuce on a serving dish. Place the cup of brown rice in the center and arrange beans on either side. Sprinkle with chopped green onions and dress with oil and vinegar or your favorite vinaigrette dressing.

2 cups cooked nonwheat
    pasta (corn, quinoa,
    or rice)
1 cup cooked chickpeas
2/3 cup chopped steamed
    broccoli
1/4 cup diced red onion
1/4 cup diced green pepper
1/2 teaspoon basil
1/2 teaspoon tarragon
3 tablespoons olive oil
juice of 1/2 lemon
1/8 teaspoon salt

Pasta with Chickpeas   *Serves 4*

Combine all ingredients in a large bowl. Mix well, chill, and serve.

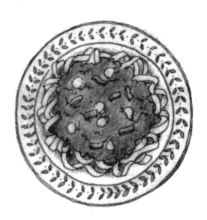

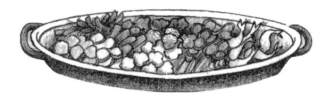

Pasta with Oil and Garlic

Serves 4

1 pound nonwheat pasta
    (rice, corn, or buckwheat)
1 clove garlic, minced
4 tablespoons flax oil
1 teaspoon basil
1/2 teaspoon sea salt
1 tablespoon soy Parmesan
    cheese (available at
    health food stores)

Cook pasta until tender. Top with garlic, flax oil, basil, salt, and soy Parmesan. Mix until well blended and serve.

Tofu and Almond Stir Fry

Serves 4

3/4 cup cubed firm tofu
1 cup raw almonds, chopped
1/4 yellow onion, chopped
1/2 red pepper, chopped
1/4 cup water
1 teaspoon sesame or saf-
    flower oil
3 cups cooked brown rice
1 teaspoon wheat-free
    (tamari) soy sauce

Combine tofu, almonds, onions, and red pepper in a large frying pan with water and oil. Cook over low flame for 5 minutes. (Add extra water to pan as needed.) Add rice to pan and mix. Heat for 5 minutes or until warm. Transfer to serving dish and toss with wheat-free soy sauce.

4 corn tortillas
3/4 pound cooked and
    pureed pinto beans
1/2 avocado, thinly sliced
1/4 sweet red pepper,
    diced
1 tomato, diced
1/4 red onion, finely
    chopped
1/2 head red or romaine
    lettuce, chopped
6 tablespoons salsa

Vegetarian Tacos   *Serves 4*

Warm tortillas and beans in separate pans. Place tortillas on individual serving dishes and spread with beans. Garnish with avocado, pepper, tomato, and onion; then cover each taco with lettuce and 1-1/2 tablespoons of salsa.

4 fillets of salmon,
    3 oz. each
1 cup water
juice of 1 lemon

Poached Salmon   *Serves 4*

Combine water and lemon juice in skillet and heat. Place salmon in the hot liquid. Cover and poach for 6 to 8 minutes or until salmon flakes easily with a fork. Remove fish and keep it warm until you are ready to serve.

4 fillets of tuna, 4 oz. each
1 tablespoon canola oil
2 tablespoons lemon juice

Broiled Tuna   *Serves 4*

Baste the tuna fillets with oil; then sprinkle with lemon juice. Place tuna in a broiler pan. Broil for 5 to 6 minutes, or until fish is done to your liking.

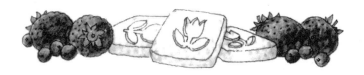

Snacks

Trail Mix *Makes 3/4 cup*

4 oz. raw unsalted pumpkin seeds

4 oz. raw unsalted sunflower seeds

4 oz. raisins

Combine and store in a container in the refrigerator. *This trail mix is very high in essential fatty acids, calcium, magnesium, and iron. I use it for a snack food to replace stressful and unhealthy sugar-based sweets and chocolate. It is a great mix to take on trips, and I eat it often for breakfast.*

Rice Cakes with Nut Butter and Jam *Serves 2*

4 unsalted rice cakes

2 tablespoons raw almond butter

2 tablespoons fruit preserves (no added sugar)

Spread rice cakes with almond butter and fruit preserves for a quick snack. *Herbal tea makes a good accompaniment.*

Rice Cakes with Tuna Fish *Serves 2*

4 unsalted rice cakes

4 oz. tuna fish

2 teaspoons low-calorie mayonnaise

Spread rice cakes with tuna fish and mayonnaise. This is an excellent high-protein, high-carbohydrate snack.

Apple with
Almond Butter   *Serves 2*

1 apple, sliced
1 tablespoon raw almond
  butter

Spread almond butter on thin
apple slices.

Banana with
Sesame Butter   *Serves 2*

1 banana, halved
1 tablespoon raw sesame
  butter

Spread sesame butter on each half
of a ripe banana.

Popcorn and Flax Oil   *Serves 2*

4 oz. popcorn
2 tablespoons flax oil
1/2 teaspoon salt substitute

Air-pop the popcorn into a large
bowl. Sprinkle with flax oil and a
salt substitute.

6

Vitamins, Minerals, Herbs, & Essential Fatty Acids

*N*utritional supplements can play an important role in the treatment and prevention of fibroids and endometriosis. Supplements can help to balance hormones and reduce estrogen levels. When used properly, they can have a dramatic effect on the regulation of bleeding and the reduction of the pain and cramps that may accompany both fibroids and endometriosis. The importance of nutrition in balancing estrogen levels and relieving excessive menstrual bleeding, cramping, and pain is supported by many medical research studies done at university centers and hospitals; a bibliography is provided at the end of this chapter for those wanting more information.

Use of supplements must go hand in hand with a low-stress, healthful diet. It is not enough to take supplements and continue with poor dietary habits. I have seen women try this and not get the results they're looking for. However, diet alone can't provide the nutrient levels necessary for optimal healing. The use of supplements can speed up and facilitate the return to vibrant health and well-being.

This chapter is divided into four sections. The first discusses the role of vitamins and minerals for treatment of fibroids and endometriosis. The second section describes which herbs are helpful for the relief of fibroid and endometriosis symptoms; the third section explains the important therapeutic role of essential fatty acids. In the fourth section, I recommend specific nutritional formulas for fibroids and endometriosis and tell how to use them. Charts toward the end of the chapter list major food sources of each essential nutrient discussed.

Vitamins and Minerals for Women with Fibroids and Endometriosis

The following vitamins and minerals play an important role in both the symptomatic relief and prevention of fibroids and endometriosis.

Vitamin A. Heavy menstrual bleeding is a significant problem for women with fibroids and is the most common reason for hysterectomies. Bleeding is also a significant problem for women with endometriosis (one-third of all endometriosis patients complain of excessive flow and spotting). Fortunately, vitamin A can play a role in reducing these symptoms.

In a study of 71 women with excessive bleeding, the women were found to have significantly lower blood levels of vitamin A than the normal population. Almost 90 percent of the women studied returned to a normal bleeding pattern after two weeks of vitamin A treatment. Vitamin A is needed for the healthy production of red blood cells; it is also necessary for the normal growth and support of the eyes, skin, mucous membranes, and healthy immune function. Deficiency of vitamin A results in impaired immune function; rough, scaly skin; and night blindness.

There are two types of vitamin A. Vitamin A from animal sources usually comes from fish liver and is oil soluble. This type of vitamin A can be toxic if taken in too large a dose (i.e., greater than 25,000 international units [I.U.] per day, if taken for more than a few months). In contrast, beta carotene, the precursor of vitamin A found in plants, is water soluble and is not toxic in large amounts. A single sweet potato or cup of carrot juice contains more than 20,000 I.U. of beta carotene.

Vitamin B Complex. The vitamin B complex consists of eleven factors that perform many important biochemical functions in the body. These include stabilization of brain chemistry, glucose metabolism, and the inactivation of estrogen by the liver. Since fibroids and endometriosis can be triggered by excess estrogen in the body, it is important that estrogen levels are properly regulated through breakdown and disposal by the liver. In pioneering animal and human research in 1942 and 1943, Biskind highlighted the important role of several B-complex vitamins in regulating estrogen levels by promoting healthy liver function. Women with several problems related to excessive estrogen levels—including heavy menstrual flow, PMS, and fibrocystic breast disease—received supplements of vitamin B complex. When supplemented with thiamine (B_1), riboflavin (B_2), niacin and niacinamide (B_3), as well as the rest of the B complex, the women in this research study showed relief of estrogen-related symptoms.

Besides helping to regulate estrogen levels, B vitamins have been found useful for the reduction of menstrual pain and cramps, particularly vitamin B_6 or pyridoxine. In clinical studies, use of B_6 led to a reduction in PMS-related cramping, fluid retention, weight gain, and fatigue. PMS often coexists with fibroids and endometriosis. An interesting clinical study done in 1978 tested the usefulness of vitamin B_6 in decreasing menstrual pain and cramps. Women received vitamin B_6 daily throughout the menstrual period as well as during the rest of the month. Duration and intensity of their cramps decreased progressively over a four- to six-month period.

Vitamin B_6 is also an important factor in the conversion of linoleic acid to gamma linolenic acid (GLA) in the production of the beneficial series-one prostaglandins. Series-one prostaglandins have a relaxant effect on uterine muscles as well as anti-inflammatory effect on various tissues. As a result they can help relieve cramps, reduce symptoms of endometriosis, and possibly help limit the spread of implants. Because vitamin B_6 levels drop in women using the birth control pill, a common treatment for both spasmodic dysmenorrhea and endometriosis, these women should take supplemental B_6. Such women safely take B_6 in doses up to 300 milligrams. Avoid doses above this level because they can be neurotoxic.

For women with fibroids and endometriosis, I generally recommend 50 to 100 milligrams per day of vitamin B complex, with additional B_6 (up to 300 milligrams total daily dose), if appropriate. The B vitamins are water soluble and easily lost from the body. In fact, emotional and nutritional stress accelerate the loss of these essential nutrients. This can worsen symptoms seen with fibroids and endometriosis, including fatigue, faintness, and dizziness. Even with supplementation, a diet high in B complex is desirable for all women. The B-complex vitamins are commonly found in whole grains, beans and peas, and liver.

Vitamin C. Vitamin C has been tested, along with bioflavonoids, as a treatment for heavy menstrual bleeding, which is commonly found in women with fibroids and endometriosis. One study showed a reduction in bleeding in 87 percent of the women participating. Vitamin C helps reduce bleeding by strengthening capillaries and preventing capillary fragility. Women who bleed excessively may eventually become iron deficient and end up with anemia. Vitamin C helps increase iron absorption from food sources such as bran, peas, seeds, nuts, and leafy green vegetables. This can help prevent iron deficiency anemia in women with heavy bleeding.

Vitamin C also helps decrease menstrual cramps and pain by permitting better flow of nutrients into the tight and contracted uterine muscle. It also facilitates the flow of waste products out of the uterus, ensuring that waste products that worsen cramping and pain, like lactic acid and carbon dioxide, are more efficiently released from the pelvic region. Vitamin C is an important antistress vitamin essential for healthy adrenal function and immune function. It may help to limit the spread of endometrial implants through stimulating immune function and limiting inflammation and scarring. Vitamin C can also help decrease the fatigue and lethargy symptoms that accompany cramps.

I recommend that women with excessive bleeding and cramps

use between 1000 to 4000 milligrams of vitamin C per day, especially when symptoms occur. Many fruits and vegetables are excellent sources of vitamin C.

Bioflavonoids. Like vitamin C, bioflavonoids (once called vitamin P) have also shown dramatic results in their ability to reduce heavy menstrual bleeding through strengthening the capillary walls; they have been studied in conjunction with vitamin C for relief of bleeding. Bioflavonoids have been used in women with bleeding due to hormonal imbalance and have been tested in women who have lost multiple pregnancies due to bleeding. In nature, bioflavonoids can often be found with vitamin C in fruits and vegetables. For example, they are found in grape skins, cherries, blackberries, and blueberries. Bioflavonoids are also abundant in citrus fruits, especially in the pulp and the white rind. They are also found in buckwheat and soybeans.

Bioflavonoids have the additional property of being weakly estrogenic and antiestrogenic, important properties for control of fibroid and endometriosis symptoms. As a result, bioflavonoid containing plants belong to a classification of estrogen-containing plants called phytoestrogens. Other estrogen-containing plants which are nonbioflavonoidal include fennel, anise, and licorice. Though these plants are estrogenic, the doses they contain are much weaker than the levels in drugs. (Bioflavonoids contain 1/50,000 the potency of a drug dose of estrogen.) Also, plant sources of estrogen can compete with estrogen precursors produced by your body for space on the binding sites of enzymes needed for estrogen production. Thus, on the one hand, bioflavonoids can act to lower estrogen levels in the body for women with fibroids and endometriosis whose symptoms are triggered by excessive estrogen. On the other hand, the weakly estrogenic effect of the bioflavonoids can help relieve symptoms such as hot flashes, night sweats, and mood swings in women who are grossly deficient in estrogen. One study, done at Loyola University Medical School in Chicago, showed that bioflavonoids help to reduce hot flashes in menopausal women.

Vitamin E. Like bioflavonoids, this essential nutrient has been used to relieve symptoms triggered by excessive estrogen levels, including PMS, fibrocystic breast disease, and breast tenderness. I have found vitamin E to be a useful part of a therapeutic program in women with heavy menstrual bleeding due to fibroids and endometriosis.

Vitamin E has also been tested in clinical studies as a treatment for menstrual cramps and pain. Taken in doses of 150 I.U. ten days premenstrual and during the first four days of the menstrual period, it helped to relieve symptoms of menstrual discomfort in approximately 70 percent of the women tested within two menstrual cycles.

Vitamin E has been studied as an alternative treatment for menopause, because it has been shown to relieve hot flashes, night sweats, mood swings, and even vaginal dryness. It is obviously a very important nutrient for women's health. The best natural sources of vitamin E are wheat germ oil, walnut oil, soybean oil, and other grain and seed oil sources. I generally recommend that women with fibroids and endometriosis use between 400 and 2000 I.U. per day. Women with hypertension and diabetes should start on a much lower dose of vitamin E (100 I.U. per day). Any increase in dosage should be made slowly and monitored carefully in these women. Otherwise, vitamin E tends to be extremely safe and is commonly used by millions of people.

Iron. Women who suffer from heavy menstrual bleeding due to fibroids and endometriosis tend to be iron deficient. In fact, some medical studies have found that inadequate iron intake may even cause excessive bleeding. Women who suffer from heavy menstrual bleeding should have their red blood count checked to see if they need supplemental iron in addition to a high-iron-content diet. Heme iron, the iron from meat sources like liver, is much better absorbed and assimilated than nonheme iron, the iron from vegetarian sources. To be absorbed properly, nonheme iron must be taken with at least 75 milligrams of vitamin C.

Iron deficiency is the main cause of anemia due to heavy menstrual flow. Iron is an essential component of red blood cells, combining with protein and copper to make hemoglobin, the pigment of the red blood cells. Iron deficiency is common during all phases of a woman's life and is a frequent cause of fatigue and low-energy states. Good food sources of iron include liver, blackstrap molasses, beans and peas, seeds and nuts, and certain fruits and vegetables.

Calcium. This important mineral helps to prevent menstrual pain and cramps by maintaining normal muscle tone. Because cramps are common with fibroids and endometriosis, calcium intake is important to help prevent further muscular irritability. When taken before bed at night, calcium is effective in helping to combat insomnia due to menstrual discomfort. Muscles that are calcium deficient tend to be hyperactive and more likely to cramp. Since the uterus is made up of muscle, it is susceptible to calcium deficiency. Besides promoting normal muscle tone and activity, calcium is a major structural component of bone. Unfortunately, calcium deficiency is common in our society. The recommended daily allowance (RDA) for calcium in menstruating women is 800 milligrams per day and rises to as much as 1500 milligrams per day in postmenopausal women. The typical American diet supplies only about 450 to 550 milligrams per day. No wonder so many American women are at risk for problems like menstrual cramps and osteoporosis. Good food sources of calcium include green leafy vegetables, beans and peas, seeds and nuts, blackstrap molasses, and seafood.

Magnesium. Magnesium has an important effect on the neuromuscular system in reducing menstrual cramps. A deficiency of magnesium increases muscular hyperactivity and can worsen menstrual pain that is already severe due to fibroids and endometriosis. Magnesium optimizes the amount of usable calcium in your system by increasing calcium absorption. Conversely, calcium can interfere with magnesium absorption. Magnesium deficiency contributes to menstrual fatigue, dizziness, and fainting because of its importance in glucose metabolism. A magnesium deficiency can hinder the normal conversion of food to usable energy. Magnesium is also needed for the conversion of linoleic acid to gamma linolenic acid (GLA), and a deficiency of magnesium retards the conversion of essential fatty acids to the series-one prostaglandins. Like calcium, magnesium is an important structural component of healthy bone tissue, necessary for the prevention of osteoporosis. It is usually recommended that the diet include half as much magnesium as calcium, or approximately 400 milligrams per day. Most women get only one-third to one-half of this amount in their daily diet, putting them at high risk for menstrual cramping and pain.

Potassium. Potassium is the third mineral, along with calcium and magnesium, that helps reduce cramps by regulating muscle contraction. Thus, adequate levels of potassium in the body are necessary to prevent worsening of menstrual cramps. Women deficient in potassium may suffer from premenstrual uterine cramping, leg cramps, and even irregular heartbeats. Potassium also plays a role in the maintenance of fluid balance and energy levels. Women low in potassium are more prone to PMS-related bloating, fatigue, and weakness. Women suffering from endometriosis-related diarrhea may lose significant amounts of potassium through watery bowel movements.

For women suffering from these symptoms, the use of a potassium supplement may be helpful. The most common dose available is a 99-milligram tablet or capsule. I generally recommend taking one to three per day for up to one week premenstrually. Potassium, however, must be used cautiously. It should be avoided by women with kidney or cardiovascular disease, because a high level of potassium can cause an irregular heartbeat in women with these problems. Also, potassium can be irritating to the intestinal tract, so it should be taken with meals.

Herbs for Women with Fibroids and Endometriosis

A wide variety of herbs can help alleviate symptoms of fibroids and endometriosis. I have used many of these herbs in my practice for years and have found them to be gentle, effective remedies for many women. I use them as a form of extended nutrition, as a way of balancing and expanding the diet and optimizing the nutritional intake. Some herbs have a hormone-balancing effect and help lower excessive estrogen levels and control heavy bleeding symptoms. Some herbs provide an additional source of essential nutrients such as calcium, magnesium, and potassium that help relieve menstrual pain and cramps. Other herbs have mild relaxant, diuretic, and anti-inflammatory properties that help relieve painful symptoms with a minimum of side effects. In this section, I describe specific herbs useful in reducing the symptoms of fibroids and endometriosis.

As mentioned in the vitamin section, bioflavonoids can help control fibroids and endometriosis. While purified bioflavonoids are available in capsule form, they are also a significant component of a wide variety of fruits and flowers. Bioflavonoids are responsible for the striking colors of many plants. Good sources of bioflavonoids include citrus fruits, hawthorn berries, bilberries, cherries, and grape skins. Bioflavonoids have also been found in red clover and in some clover strains in Australia. Many of these plants are available as herbal tinctures (liquid) or in capsules.

Two herbs that women traditionally used to stop excessive menstrual flow and postpartum hemorrhage are goldenseal and shepherd's purse. Recent research studies have supported the traditional claims made for these herbs. Goldenseal contains a chemical called berberine that calms uterine muscular tension. It has also been used to calm and soothe the digestive tract. Shepherd's purse promotes blood clotting and has been used to help stop menstrual bleeding. If your bleeding is excessive or irregular, consult your physician. This condition should be evaluated carefully by your physician and, if necessary, medical therapy should be instituted. Excessive and irregular bleeding can be dangerous and should never be allowed to continue without medical help. For those women for whom the menstrual flow is normal but somewhat heavier than usual, the mild properties of herbs may help relieve symptoms.

Other herbs help to prevent anemia by providing good sources of nonheme iron. Excellent examples are yellow dock and pau d'arco. Yellow dock is also used to promote liver health—an important factor in decreasing heavy bleeding through regulation of excessive estrogen levels, since the liver breaks down estrogen and prepares it for excretion from the body. Turmeric, or curcumin, is also used to promote liver health in traditional medicine. Recent research suggests that it has antibacterial properties. Turmeric is a delicious herb often used for flavoring in traditional Indian dishes. Silymarin, or milk thistle, protects liver functions through its flavonoid content. These flavonoids are strong antioxidants and help protect the liver from damage.

Anti-inflammatory Herbs. Several anti-inflammatory herbs may help relieve symptoms of endometriosis and reduce inflammation of implants. White willow has a long and distinguished history as an effective pain reliever in both the Oriental and Western healing traditions. The active painkilling chemical in white willow bark is salicin, first isolated around 1828 by French and German chemists. Years later, salicylic acid, the precursor of aspirin, was purified from this plant. Another natural source of this aspirin precursor was discovered a short time later in the herb meadowsweet. Both meadowsweet and white willow bark reduce inflammation, pain, and fever. They help treat primary menstrual cramps and menstrual headaches as well as the pain symptoms due to endometriosis, because they suppress the action of F_2 Alpha prostaglandins. Unfortunately, like aspirin, they can produce the unwanted side effects of gastric indigestion, nausea, and diarrhea, so use these herbs carefully.

Essential Fatty Acids for Women with Fibroids and Endometriosis

Sufficient essential fatty acids are an extremely important part of the nutritional program for any women with menstrual cramps caused by endometriosis or fibroid tumors. As mentioned earlier in the book, fatty acids are the raw materials from which the beneficial hormonelike chemicals called prostaglandins are made. The prostaglandins from essential fatty acids have muscle-relaxant and blood-vessel-relaxant properties that can significantly reduce muscle cramps and tension. They also have an anti-inflammatory effect on tissues that is very important in limiting this deleterious response within the endometrial implants, thereby limiting painful pelvic symptoms.

There are two essential fatty acids, linoleic acid (Omega 6 family) and linolenic acid (Omega 3 family). They are derived from specific food sources in our diets, primarily raw seeds, nuts, and certain fish such as salmon, mackerel, and trout. Unlike the unhealthy saturated fats, these fats cannot be made by the body and must be supplied daily in our diets, through either food or supplements.

Even when these fatty acids are supplied in the diet, some women lack the ability to convert them efficiently to the muscle-relaxant prostaglandins. This is particularly true with linoleic acid, which must be converted to a chemical called gamma linolenic acid (GLA) on its way to becoming the series-one prostaglandin called E_1. The conversion of linoleic acid to GLA, followed by the chemical steps leading to the creation of the beneficial prostaglandins, requires the presence of magnesium, vitamin B_6, zinc, vitamin C, and niacin. Women who are deficient in these nutrients can't make the chemical conversions effectively.

In addition, women who eat a high-cholesterol diet, eat processed oils like mayonnaise, use a great deal of alcohol, or are diabetic may have difficulty converting fatty acids to series-one prostaglandins. Other factors that impede prostaglandin production include emotional stress, allergies, and eczema. In women with these risk factors, less than one percent of linoleic acid may be converted to GLA. The rest of the fatty acids can be used as an energy source, but they will not be able to play a role in relieving menstrual pain, cramp symptoms, and inflammation due to endometriosis.

A number of interesting studies have been done on essential fatty acids as a treatment for PMS. This is particularly relevant for women suffering from fibroids and endometriosis because PMS often accompanies these problems. Women with PMS often have the congestive type of menstrual cramps with bloating, weight gain, and dull aching pain in the pelvic region. Clinical studies have shown that the use of essential fatty acids can reduce most PMS symptoms by as much as 70 percent. Evening primrose oil, borage oil, and black currant oil are the most common supplemental sources of essential fatty acids for the treatment of menstrual cramps and PMS. All three oils contain high levels of GLA, allowing women to circumvent the difficult conversion process of linoleic acid to GLA.

The best food sources of essential fatty acids are raw flax seed oil and pumpkin seed oil, which contain high levels of both linoleic acid and linolenic acid, in combination. Both the seeds and their pressed oils should be used absolutely fresh and unspoiled. Because these oils become rancid very easily when exposed to light and air (oxygen), they need to be packed in opaque containers and kept in the refrigerator. They can also be taken in capsule form.

Fresh flax seed oil—golden, rich, and delicious—is my special favorite. Good quality flax seed oil is available in health food stores. Flax seeds are particularly useful for women with fibroids and endometriosis. This is because both the flax oil and the lignans (celluloselike structure of the flax seed) are estrogenic. As with other weak dietary sources of estrogen, they help to regulate the levels of this hormone in your body. Pumpkin seed oil has a deep green color and spicy flavor; it is probably more difficult to find than flax seed oil. A good source of this oil is fresh raw pumpkin seeds.

Linolenic acid (Omega 3 family) by itself is also found in abundance in fish oils. The best sources are cold-water, high-fat fish such as salmon, tuna, rainbow trout, mackerel, and eel. Linoleic acid (Omega 6 family) by itself can be found in seeds and seed oils. Good sources include safflower oil, sunflower oil, corn oil, sesame seed oil, and wheat germ oil. Many women prefer to use raw fresh sesame seeds, sunflower seeds, and wheat germ to obtain the oils. The average healthy adult requires only four teaspoons per day of the essential oils, although women with menstrual cramps may need several tablespoons per day. If you use whole flax seed, remember that the seeds are 50 percent oil by content, so you need twice as much whole seed intake as oil for the same amount of fatty acids. For optimal results, be sure to use these oils along with vitamin E. The vitamin E also helps to prevent rancidity of the oils.

Nutritional Supplements for Women with Fibroids and Endometriosis

Good dietary habits are crucial for control of your fibroid or endometriosis symptoms. But for many women, the use of nutritional supplements is important in order to achieve high levels of certain essential nutrients. On the following pages are two formulas, a vitamin and mineral formula and an herbal formula, typical of those that I have used for many years with my patients. You can put these formulas together yourself by combining the individual nutrients in the amounts specified. The vitamin and mineral formula is also available from *The LIFE-CYCLES Center* as the Menopause Nutritional System. It provides excellent nutritional support for women during their premenopausal years, when fibroid and endometriosis symptoms can be at their worst. It also provides important nutritional support for younger women with these problems. The menopause herbal formula is also helpful for hormonal balancing in women with fibroids and endometriosis. Women with anemia due to heavy menstrual flow may want to try my iron formula, also available through *The LIFECYCLES Center*.

Remember that all women differ somewhat in their nutritional needs. If you do take the recommended vitamin or herbal supplements, I usually advise that you start with one-fourth to one-half the dose recommended in this book and work your way up slowly to the higher dosage, if needed. You may find that you do best with slightly more or less of certain ingredients.

I have found that most women can take smaller doses during the times when they are symptom-free. Two to three pills per day of my menopause formulas may be enough during the first half of your cycle. During the second half of the cycle when your symptoms worsen, you might double that dose. If you know very accurately when your symptoms will begin, you might increase the dose of the supplement a few days ahead. Do not exceed six to eight capsules per day without the supervision of your physician.

I recommend that patients take their supplements with meals or at least a snack. Very rarely, a woman will have a digestive reaction to supplements, such as nausea or indigestion. If this happens, stop all supplements; then resume using them, adding one at a time, until you find the offending nutrient. Eliminate from your program any nutrient to which you have a reaction. If you have any specific questions, ask a health-care professional who is knowledgeable about nutrition.

Optimal Nutritional Supplementation
for Fibroids and Endometriosis (Menopause Formulas)

VITAMINS AND MINERALS	Maximum Daily Dose
Vitamin A	5000 I.U.
Beta carotene (provitamin A)	5000 I.U.
Vitamin B complex	
B_1 (thiamine)	50 mg
B_2 (riboflavin)	50 mg
B_3 (niacinamide)	50 mg
B_5 (pantothenic acid)	50 mg
B_6 (pyridoxine)	30 mg
B_{12} (cyanocobalamin)	50 mcg
Folic acid	400 mcg
Biotin	200 mcg
Choline	50 mcg
Inositol	50 mg
PABA	50 mg

Vitamin C (as ascorbic acid)	1000 mg
Vitamin D	400 I.U.
Bioflavonoids	800 mg
Rutin	200 mg
Vitamin E (d-alpha tocopherol acetate)	800 I.U.
Calcium	1200 mg
Magnesium	320 mg
Potassium	100 mg
Iron	27 mg
Zinc	15 mg
Iodine	150 mcg
Manganese	10 mg
Copper	2 mg
Selenium	25 mcg
Chromium	100 mcg
Bromelain	100 mcg
Papain	65 mg
Boron	3 mg

Use two to eight tablets per day.

HERBS	*Maximum Daily Dose*
Blue cohosh	100 mg
False unicorn root	100 mg
Fennel	100 mg
Anise	100 mg
Blessed thistle	100 mg

Use one to two capsules per day.

ADDITIONAL HERBS	*Maximum Daily Dose*
White willow bark	500 mg
Yellow dock	500 mg

Use one capsule per day.

Women's Daily Iron Formula

VITAMINS AND MINERALS	*Maximum Daily Dose*
Iron	27 mg
Vitamin C	250 mg
Vitamin E (natural d-alpha)	30 I.U.
Vitamin B complex	
B_1 (thiamine)	7.5 mg
B_2 (riboflavin)	7.5 mg
B_6 (pyridoxine)	30 mg
B_5 (pantothenic acid)	50 mg
B_3 (niacinamide)	10 mg
B_{12} (cyanocobalamin)	250 mcg
Folic acid	400 mcg
Biotin	100 mcg
Choline bitartrate	5 mg
Inositol	5 mg
PABA	5 mg
Zinc	1.5 mg
Copper	250 mcg
Betaine HCL	10 mg
Chlorophyll	35 mg
Licorice root	25 mg
Red clover	25 mg
Yellow dock	25 mg

Use one capsule per day.

Food Sources of Vitamin A

Vegetables	*Fruits*	*Meat, poultry, seafood*
Carrots	Apricots	Crab
Carrot juice	Avocado	Halibut
Collard greens	Cantaloupe	Liver—all types
Dandelion greens	Mangoes	Mackerel
Green onions	Papaya	Salmon
Kale	Peaches	Swordfish
Parsley	Persimmons	
Spinach		
Sweet potatoes		
Turnip greens		
Winter squash		

Food Sources of Vitamin B Complex (including folic acid)

Vegetables	*Legumes*	*Grains*
Alfalfa	Garbanzo beans	Barley
Artichoke	Lentils	Bran
Asparagus	Lima beans	Brown rice
Beets	Pinto beans	Corn
Broccoli	Soybeans	Millet
Brussels sprouts		Rice bran
Cabbage	*Meat, poultry,*	Wheat
Cauliflower	*seafood*	Wheat germ
Green beans	Egg yolks*	
Kale	Liver*	*Sweeteners*
Leeks		Blackstrap molasses
Onions		
Peas		
Romaine lettuce		

Eggs and meat should be from organic, range-fed stock fed on pesticide-free food.

Food Sources of Vitamin B$_6$

Grains	Vegetables	Meat, poultry, seafood
Brown rice	Asparagus	Chicken
Buckwheat flour	Beet greens	Salmon
Rice bran	Broccoli	Shrimp
Rice polishings	Brussels sprouts	Tuna
Rye flour	Cauliflower	
Wheat germ	Green peas	*Nuts and seeds*
Whole wheat flour	Leeks	Sunflower seeds
	Sweet potatoes	

Food Sources of Vitamin C

Fruits	Vegetables and legumes	Meat, poultry, seafood
Blackberries	Asparagus	Liver—all types
Black currants	Black-eyed peas	Pheasant
Cantaloupe	Broccoli	Quail
Elderberries	Brussels sprouts	Salmon
Grapefruit	Cabbage	
Grapefruit juice	Cauliflower	
Guavas	Collards	
Kiwi fruit	Green onions	
Mangoes	Green peas	
Oranges	Kale	
Orange juice	Kohlrabi	
Pineapple	Parsley	
Raspberries	Potatoes	
Strawberries	Rutabagas	
Tangerines	Sweet pepper	
Tomatoes	Sweet potatoes	
	Turnips	

Food Sources of Vitamin E

Vegetables	*Meats, poultry,*	*Grains*
Asparagus	*seafood*	Brown rice
Cucumber	Haddock	Millet
Green peas	Herring	
Kale	Mackerel	*Fruits*
	Lamb	Mangoes
Nuts and seeds	Liver—all types	
Almonds		
Brazil nuts	*Oils*	
Hazelnuts	Corn oil	
Peanuts	Peanut oil	
	Safflower oil	
	Sesame oil	
	Soybean oil	
	Wheat germ oil	

Food Sources of Essential Fatty Acids

Flax oil
Pumpkin oil
Soybean oil
Walnut oil
Safflower oil
Sunflower oil
Grape oil
Corn oil
Wheat germ oil
Sesame oil

Food Sources of Iron

Grains	Vegetables	Meat, poultry, seafood
Bran cereal (All-Bran)	Beets	
Bran muffin	Beet greens	Beef liver
Millet, dry	Broccoli	Calf's liver
Oat flakes	Brussels sprouts	Chicken liver
Pasta, whole wheat	Corn	Clams
Pumpernickel bread	Dandelion greens	Oysters
Wheat germ	Green beans	Sardines
	Kale	Scallops
Legumes	Leeks	Trout
Black beans	Spinach	
Black-eyed peas	Sweet potatoes	Nuts and seeds
Garbanzo beans	Swiss chard	Almonds
Kidney beans		Pecans
Lentils	Fruits	Pistachios
Lima beans	Apple juice	Sesame butter
Pinto beans	Avocado	Sesame seeds
Soybeans	Blackberries	Sunflower seeds
Split peas	Dates, dried	
Tofu	Figs	
	Prunes, dried	
	Prune juice	
	Raisins	

Food Sources of Calcium

Vegetables and legumes	Meat, poultry, seafood	Fruits
Artichoke	Abalone	Blackberries
Black beans	Beef	Black currants
Black-eyed peas	Bluefish	Boysenberries
Beet greens	Carp	Oranges
Broccoli	Crab	Pineapple juice
Brussels sprouts	Haddock	Prunes
Cabbage	Herring	Raisins
Collards	Lamb	Rhubarb
Eggplant	Lobster	Tangerine juice
Garbanzo beans	Oysters	*Grains*
Green beans	Perch	Bran
Green onions	Salmon	Brown rice
Kale	Shrimp	Bulgar wheat
Kidney beans	Venison	Millet
Leeks		
Lentils		
Parsley		
Parsnips		
Pinto beans		
Rutabagas		
Soybeans		
Spinach		
Turnips		
Watercress		

Food Sources of Magnesium

Vegetables and legumes	Meat, poultry, seafood	Nuts and seeds
Artichoke	Beef	Almonds
Black-eyed peas	Carp	Brazil nuts
Carrot juice	Chicken	Hazelnuts
Corn	Clams	Peanuts
Green peas	Cod	Pistachios
Leeks	Crab	Pumpkin seeds
Lima beans	Duck	Sesame seeds
Okra	Haddock	Walnuts
Parsnips	Herring	
Potatoes	Lamb	*Fruits*
Soybean sprouts	Mackerel	Avocado
Spinach	Oysters	Banana
Squash	Salmon	Grapefruit juice
Yams	Shrimp	Pineapple juice
	Snapper	Raisins
	Turkey	Prunes
		Papaya
		Grains
		Millet
		Brown rice
		Wild rice

Food Sources of Potassium

Vegetables and legumes	Meat, poultry, seafood	Nuts and seeds
Artichoke	Bass	Almonds
Asparagus	Beef	Brazil nuts
Black-eyed peas	Carp	Chestnuts
Beets	Catfish	Hazelnuts
Brussels sprouts	Chicken	Macadamia nuts
Carrot juice	Cod	Peanuts
Cauliflower	Duck	Pistachios
Corn	Eel	Pumpkin seeds
Garbanzo beans	Flatfish	Sesame seeds
Green beans	Haddock	Sunflower seeds
Kidney beans	Halibut	Walnuts
Leeks	Herring	
Lentils	Lamb	*Fruits*
Lima beans	Lobster	Apricots
Navy beans	Mackerel	Avocado
Okra	Oysters	Banana
Parsnips	Perch	Cantaloupe
Peas	Pike	Currants
Pinto beans	Salmon	Figs
Potatoes	Scallops	Grapefruit juice
Pumpkin	Shrimp	Orange juice
Soybean sprouts	Snapper	Papaya
Spinach	Trout	Pineapple juice
Squash	Turkey	Prunes
Yams		Raisins

Grains
Brown rice
Millet
Wild rice

Suggested Reading

Castleman, M. *The Healing Herbs.* Emmaus, PA: Rodale Press, 1991.

Erasmus, U. *Fats and Oils.* Burnaby, BC, Canada: Alive Books, 1986.

Gittleman, A. L. *Supernutrition for Women.* New York: Bantam Books, 1991.

Hasslering, B., S. Greenwood, M.D., and M. Castleman. *The Medical Self-Care Book of Women's Health.* New York: Doubleday, 1987.

Hogladaroom, G., R. McCorkle, and N. Woods. *The Complete Book of Women's Health.* Englewood Cliffs, NJ: Prentice-Hall, 1982.

Kirschmann, J., and L. Dunne. *Nutrition Almanac.* New York: McGraw-Hill, 1984.

Kutsky, R. *Vitamins and Hormones.* New York: Van Nostrand Reinhold, 1973.

Lambert-Lagace, L. *The Nutrition Challenge for Women.* Palo Alto, CA: Bull Publishing, 1990.

Lark, S., M.D. *Anemia and Heavy Menstrual Flow: A Self-Help Program.* Los Altos, CA: Westchester Publishing, 1992.

Lark, S., M.D. *Menopause Self-Help Book.* Berkeley, CA: Celestial Arts, 1990.

Lark, S., M.D. *Menstrual Cramps: A Self-Help Program.* Los Altos, CA: Westchester Publishing, 1992.

Lark, S., M.D. *Premenstrual Syndrome Self-Help Book.* Berkeley, CA: Celestial Arts, 1984.

Lauerson, N. *The Endometriosis Answer Book.* New York: Fowlett Columbine, 1989.

Mowrey, D., Ph.D. *The Scientific Validation of Herbal Medicine.* New Canaan, CT: Keats Publishing, 1986.

Murray, M., N.D. *The 21st Century Herbal.* Bellevue, WA: Vita-Line, Inc., 1992.

Padus, E. *The Woman's Encyclopedia of Health and Natural Healing.* Emmaus, PA: Rodale Press, 1981.

Reuben, C., and J. Priestly. *Essential Supplements for Women.* New York: Perigree Books, 1988.

Articles

Abraham, G. E. Primary dysmenorrhea. *Clinical Obstetrics and Gynecology* 1978; 21(1):139–45.

Abraham , G. E. Magnesium deficiency in premenstrual tension. *Magnesium Bulletin* 1982; 1:68–73.

Abraham, G. E. Premenstrual tension syndromes: A nutritional approach. *Anabolism* 1986; 5(2):5–6.

Biskind, M. S., and G. R. Biskind. Effect of vitamin B complex deficiency on inactivation of estrone in the liver. *Endocrinology* 1942; 31:109–114.

Biskind, M. S. Nutritional deficiency in the etiology of menorrhagia, cystic mastitis and premenstrual tension, treatment with vitamin B complex. *Journal of Clinical Endocrinology and Metabolism* 1943; 3:227–34.

Bulbrook, P. D., J. L. Haywar, and C. Spicer. Relationship between urinary androgen and corticoid excretion and subsequent breast cancer. *Lancet* 1971; 2:395.

Butler, E. B., and E. McKnight. Vitamin E in the treatment of primary dysmenorrhea. *Lancet* 1955; 1:844–47.

Cheng, E. W., et al. Estrogenic activity of some naturally occurring isoflavones. *Annals of New York Academy of Sciences* 1955; 61(3):652.

Clemetson, C. A. B., et al. Capillary strength and the menstrual cycle. *New York Academy of Sciences* 1962; 93(7):277.

Cohen, J. D., and H. W. Rubin. Functional menorrhagia: Treatment with bioflavonoids and vitamin C. *Current Therapeutic Research* 1960; 2(11):539.

Dickinson, L. F., et al. Estrogen profiles of oriental and caucasian women in Hawaii. *New England Journal of Medicine* 1971; 291: 1211–13.

Farley, P., M.D., and J. Foland, M.D. Iron deficiency anemia: How to diagnose and correct. *Postgraduate Medicine* 1990; 87(2):89–101.

Follingstad, A. R. Commentary: Estriol the forgotten estrogen? *Journal of the American Medical Association* 1978; 239(1):29–30.

Fontana-Klaider, H., and B. Hogg. Therapeutic effects of magnesium in dysmenorrhea. *Schweiz Rundsch Med Prax* 1990; 17:79(16):491–4.

Forman, A., U. Ulmsten, and K. E. Andersson. Aspects of inhibition of myometrial hyperactivity in primary dysmenorrhea. *Acta Obstetrica et Gynecologica Scandinavica* 1983; 113:71–76.

Forster, H. B., H. Niklas, and S. Lutz. Antispasmodic effect of some medicinal plants. *Planta Medica* 1980; 40:309–19.

Glen, I., et al. The role of essential fatty acids in alcohol dependence and tissue damage. *Alcoholism* (NY) 1987; 11(1):37.

Golden, B. R., et al. Effect of diet on excretion of estrogens in pre- and post-menopausal women. *Cancer Research* 1981; 41:3771–73.

Golden, B. R., et al. Estrogen excretion patterns and plasma levels in vegetarian and omnivorous women. *New England Journal of Medicine* 1982; 307:1542–47.

Goodnight, S. H. The effects of Omega-3 fatty acids on thrombosis and atherogenesis. *Hematologic Pathology* 1989; 3(1):1.

Gugliano, D., and R. Torella. Prostaglandin E_1 inhibits glucose-induced insulin secretion in man. *Prostaglandins and Medicine* 1979; 48:302.

Hanset, A. E., et al. Eczema and essential fatty acids. *American Journal of Disease of Children* 1947; 73:1.

Harris, C. The vicious cycle of anemia and menorrhagia. *Canadian Medical Association Journal* 1957; 77:98.

Hernell, Q., et al. Suspected faulty essential fatty acid metabolism in Sjogren-Larrson Syndrome. *Pediatric Research* 1982; 16:45.

Hikino, H. Recent research on Oriental medicinal plants. *Economic Medicinal Plant Research* 1985; 1:53–86.

Hill, M. J., et al. Gut bacteria and aetiology of cancer of the breast. *Lancet* 1971; 2:472–73.

Hodges, R. E., et al. Hematopoietic studies in vitamin A deficiency. *American Journal of Clinical Nutrition* 1978; 31:876–85.

Hollander, D., and A. Tarmawski. Dietary essential fatty acids and the decline in peptic ulcer disease. *Gut* 1986; 22(3):239.

Horrobin, D. F. A biochemical basis for alcoholism and alcohol-induced damage including the fetal alcohol syndrome and cirrhosis: Interference with essential fatty acid and prostaglandin metabolism. *Medical Hypothese* 1980; 6(9):929.

Horrobin, D. F. Essential fatty acid and prostaglandin metabolism in Sjogren's Syndrome, systemic sclerosis and rheumatoid arthritis. *Scandinavian Journal of Rheumatology Supplement* 1980; 61:242.

Horrobin, D. F. Essential fatty acids and the complications of diabetes mellitus. *Wien Klin Wochenschur* 1989; 101(8):289.

Horrobin, D. F. Essential fatty acids in clinical dermatology. *Journal of the American Academy of Dermatology* 1987; 20(6):1045.

Horrobin, D. F. The regulation of prostaglandin biosynthesis by the manipulation of essential fatty acid metabolism. *Revue of Pure and Applied Pharmacologic Science* 1980; 4(4):339.

Horrobin, D. F. The role of essential fatty acids and prostaglandins in the premenstrual syndrome. *Journal of Reproductive Medicine* 1983; 28(7):465.

Hudgins, A. P. Vitamins P, C and niacin for dysmenorrhea therapy. *Western Journal of Surgery and Gynecology* 1954; 62:610–11.

Hunt, J. R., et al. Ascorbic acid: Effect on ongoing iron absorption and status in iron-depleted young women. *American Journal of Clinical Nutrition* 1990; 51:649–55.

Kappas, A., et al. Nutrition-endocrine interactions: Induction of reciprocal changes in the Δ^4- 5a-reduction of testosterone and the cytochrome p-450-dependent oxidation of estradiol by dietary macronutrients in man. *Proceedings of the National Academy of Sciences* 1983; 80:7646–49.

Kellis, T., and L. E. Vickery. Inhibition of human estrogen synthetase (aromatase) by flavones. *Science* 1984; 225:1032–34.

Kryzhanovski, G. N., N. L. Luzina, and K. N. Iarygin. Alpha-tocopherol induced activation of the endogenous opioid system. *Biull Eksp Biol Med* 1989; 108(11):566–67.

Kryzhanovski, G. N., L. P. Bakuleva, N. L. Luzina, V. A. Vinogradov, and K. N. Iarygin. Endogenous opioid system in the realization of the analgesic effect of alpha-tocopherol in reference to algomenorrhea. *Biull Eksp Biol Med* 1988; 105(2):148–50.

Lithgow, P. M., and W. M. Politzer. Vitamin A in the treatment of menorrhagia. *South African Medical Journal* 1977; 51:191.

London, R. S., et al. Mammary dysplasia: Clinical response and urinary excretion of 11-desoxy-17-ketosteroids and pregnanediol following alpha-tocopherol therapy. *Breast* 1978; 4:19.

London, R. S., et al. Endocrine parameters and alpha-tocopherol therapy of patients with mammary dysplasia. *Cancer Research* 1981; 41:3811.

London, R. S., et al. The effect of alpha-tocopherol on premenstrual symptomatology: A double-blind trial. *Journal of the American College of Nutrition* 1983; 2:115–22.

Luzina, N. L., and L. P. Vakuleva. Use of an antioxidant, alpha-tocopherol acetate, in the complex treatment of algomenorrhea. *Akush Ginekol (Mosk)* 1987; May(5):67–69.

MacMahon, B., et al. Urine oestrogen profiles of Asian and North American women. *International Journal of Cancer* 1974; 4:161–67.

Mieli-Fournial, A. Trace elements in the treatment of dysmenorrhea. *Bulletin de la Federation des Societes de Gynecologic et d'Obstetrique de Langue Francaise* 1968; 20(5):432–33.

Miscizynz, G., et al. Gallstones and Uterine Fibroids. *Surgery, Gynecology and Obstetrics* 1987; 11, Vol. 165:429–34.

Monsen, E. R. Ascorbic acid: An enhancing factor in iron absorption. *Nutritional Bioavailability of Iron.* American Chemical Society 1982; 85–95.

Pearse, H. A., and J. D. Trisler. A rational approach to the treatment of habitual abortion and menometrorrhagia. *Clinical Medicine* 1957; 9:1081.

Petkov, V. Plants with hypotensive, antiatheromatous and coronaroldilating action. *American Journal of Clinical Medicine* 1979; 7:197–236.

Pope, G. S., et al. Isolation of an oestrogenic isoflavone (biochanin A) from red clover. *Chemistry and Industry* 1953; 10:1042.

Preuter, G. W. A treatment for excessive uterine bleeding. *Applied Therapeutics* 1961; 5:351.

Puolakka, J., et al. Biochemical and clinical effects of treating the premenstrual syndrome with prostaglandin synthesis precursors. *Journal of Reproductive Medicine* 1985; 39(3):149–53.

Roberts, H. J. Perspective on vitamin E as therapy. *Journal of the American Medical Association* 1981; 246:129.

Schwartz, A. G. Inhibition of spontaneous breast cancer formation in female C3H-AVY/A mice by long-term treatment with dehydroepiandrosterone. *Cancer Research* 1979; 39:1129.

Seifert, B., P. Wagler, S. Dartsch, U. Schmidt, and J. Nieder. Magnesium—a new therapeutic alternative in primary dysmenorrhea. *Zentralbl Gynakol* 1989; 111(11):755–60.

Seltzer, S. Pain relief by dietary manipulation and tryptophan supplements. *Journal of Endodontics* 1985; 11:449–53.

Shafer, N. Iron in the treatment of dysmenorrhea: A preliminary report. *Current Therapy Research* 1965; 7:365–66.

Soloman, D., et al. Relationship between vitamin E and urinary excretion of ketosteroid fractions in cystic mastitis. *Annals of New York Academy of Science* 1972; 203:103.

Sundaram, G. S., et al. Alpha tocopherol and serum lipoproteins. *Lipids* 1981; 16:223.

Sundaram, G. S., et al. Serum hormones and lipoproteins in benign breast disease. *Cancer Research* 1981; 41:3814

Tant, D. Megaloblastic anemia due to pyridoxine deficiency associated with prolonged ingestion of an estrogen-containing oral contraceptive. *British Medical Journal* October 23, 1976; 979.

Taylor, F. A. Habitual abortion: Therapeutic evaluation of citrus bioflavonoids. *Western Journal of Surgery, Obstetrics and Gynecology* 1956; 5:280.

Taymor, M. L., et al. The etiological role of chronic iron deficiency in production of menorrhagia. *Journal of the American Medical Association* 1964; 187:323.

Taymor, M. L., et al. Menorrhagia due to chronic iron deficiency. *Obstetrics and Gynecology* 1960; 16:571.

Wang, D. Y., and M. Herrian. Plasma dehydroepiandrosterone SO_4 and breast cancer. *Acta Endocrinologica Supplementation* 1973; 177:30.

Wilcox, G., et al. Estrogen effects of plant foods in postmenopausal women. *British Medical Journal* 1990; 301:905–6.

7

Stress Reduction for Relief of Fibroids & Endometriosis

*M*any of the fibroid and endometriosis patients I see in my medical practice complain of major stress along with their physical symptoms. My personal impression as a physician who has worked with women patients for close to 20 years is that stress is a significant component of many recurrent and chronic health problems, including fibroids and endometriosis. To discount the effects of lifestyle stress on illness is a grave mistake. If the physician ignores stress as a contributing factor, the patient never receives the tools or insight necessary to modify her habits and behavior to better support good health and well-being.

Research studies have confirmed the negative effects of stress on many different diseases. On the physiological level, stress increases the cortisone output from the adrenal glands, impairs immune function, elevates blood pressure and heart rate, and affects hormonal balance. In women with fibroids and endometriosis, stress may negatively affect hormonal balance and muscle tone, upsetting the estrogen and progesterone balance and triggering excessive output of adrenal stress hormones. This can impair the body's ability to limit the scarring and inflammation caused by the endometrial implants. Growth in the size of fibroid tumors is also seen during times of stress.

Stress in fibroid and endometriosis patients can arise over such issues as job security and performance, money worries, relationship problems with family and friends, overwork, and a host of other common problems. In addition, women with fibroids and endometriosis have specific stress due to the diseases themselves, including concerns about their health and about the painful symptoms that are disrupting their lives and well-being. The infertility that can result from fibroids and endometriosis is a particularly upsetting problem for women who are trying to start a family. The pain during intercourse that is also common in women with endometriosis can disrupt a healthy sexual relationship, causing anguish and discord.

A variety of stress management techniques can help women suffering from fibroids and endometriosis. Some women find counseling or psychotherapy to be effective, while others depend heavily on the support of family and friends. Many women find it helpful to rethink their way of handling stressful situations and to implement lifestyle changes. Practicing stress-reduction techniques like meditation and deep-breathing exercises on a regular basis also helps them handle stress more effectively, as does a program of physical exercise. Whatever methods you decide to practice, I urge you to look at your stress level carefully and make every effort to handle emotionally-charged issues as calmly as possible.

The stress management exercises described in this chapter are a very important part of the fibroid and endometriosis self-help program I recommend to my patients. For many women, the intensity of menstrual pain and cramps varies from month to month, depending on many lifestyle factors. My patients frequently tell me their bleeding and cramps are worse when they are more upset. As you begin to anticipate the onset of your menstrual period, I recommend using stress-reduction techniques on a daily basis. They can really make a difference. If you break up the tasks of the day with a few minutes of stress-reducing exercises, you will feel much more relaxed. With the use of these stress-reduction techniques, you can accomplish tasks on time but in a much more relaxed, enjoyable, and health-enhancing manner.

Exercises for Relaxation

To help you cope with the emotional stresses that may become magnified if you are suffering from fibroid- and endometriosis-related symptoms, I recommend a variety of relaxation methods. Focusing, meditation, muscle relaxation, affirmations, and visualizations can each help foster a sense of calm and well-being if practiced on a regular basis. This chapter includes exercises from all of these categories for you to try. Pick those you enjoy most and practice them on a regular basis. I have taught these exercises to women patients for many years and love to practice them myself. Sometimes I recommend that my patients learn these techniques on their own through books and tapes; other times I teach the exercises to patients at my office. My patients have been very enthusiastic about the results they attain through stress-reduction exercises. They often tell me that they feel much calmer and happier. They also find their physical health improves. A calm mind seems to have beneficial effects on the body's physiology and chemistry, restoring the body to a normal condition.

To prepare yourself for the relaxation exercises in this chapter, I suggest taking the following steps:

First Step. Wear loose, comfortable clothes. Find a comfortable position. For many women, this means lying on their backs. You may also do the exercises sitting up. Try to make your spine as straight as possible. Uncross your arms and legs.

Second Step. Focus your attention on the exercises. Do not allow distracting thoughts to interfere with your concentration. Close your eyes and take a few deep breaths, in and out. This will help remove your thoughts from the problems and tasks of the day and begin to quiet your mind.

Exercise 1: Focusing

If you have fibroid- or endometriosis-related menstrual cramps and pelvic pain, this focusing exercise takes your attention off your pelvic region and lower part of your body as you focus elsewhere, clearing your mind and breathing deeply. At the end of this exercise, you may find that your discomfort is less severe. This is also a helpful exercise for inducing a sense of peace and calm.

- Sit upright in a comfortable position.

- Hold your watch in the palm of your hand.

- Focus all of your attention on the movements of the second hand of the watch.

- Inhale and exhale as you do this. Continue to concentrate for 30 seconds. Don't let any other thoughts enter your mind. At the end of this time, notice your breathing. You will probably find that it has slowed down and is calmer. You may also feel a sense of peacefulness and a decrease in any anxiety that you had on beginning this exercise.

Exercise 2: Peaceful Meditation

Many women suffering from fibroids or endometriosis complain of daily life stresses. Stress can lower the pain threshold, increasing muscle tension and discomfort. It can also worsen PMS-related irritability and mood swings, which often coexist with fibroids and endometriosis. Simple meditation techniques are a way to combat this stress.

Meditation requires you to sit quietly and engage in a simple and repetitive activity. By emptying your mind, you give yourself a rest. The metabolism of your body slows down. Meditating gives your mind a break from tension and worry. It is particularly useful during menstruation, when every little stress is magnified. After meditating you may find your mood greatly improved and your ability to handle everyday stress enhanced.

- Lie or sit in a comfortable position.

- Close your eyes and breathe deeply. Let your breathing be slow and relaxed.

- Focus all of your attention on your breathing. Notice the movement of your chest and abdomen in and out.

- Block out all other thoughts, feelings, and sensations. If you feel your attention wandering, bring it back to your breathing.

- Say the word "rest" as you inhale. Say the word "relax" as you exhale. Draw out the pronunciation of each word so that it lasts for the entire breath: r-r-r-r-e-e-e-e-s-s-s-s-t-t-t-t, r-r-r-e-e-e-l-l-l-a-a-a-x-x-x. Repeating these two words will help you to concentrate.

- Repeat this exercise until you feel very relaxed.

Exercise 3: Healing Meditation

This meditation exercise promotes healing through a series of beautiful and peaceful images you can invoke to create a positive mental state during your premenstrual and menstrual time of the month. (You can use this exercise during your symptom-free time, too.)

The premise of a healing meditation is the fact that the mind and body are inextricably linked. When you visualize a beautiful scene in which your body is being healed, you stimulate positive chemical and hormonal changes that help to create this condition. This process can reduce pain, discomfort, and irritability. Likewise, if you visualize a negative scene, such as a fight with a spouse or a boss, the negative mental picture can trigger an output of chemicals in the body that can worsen the symptoms caused by fibroids or endometriosis. The axiom "you are what you think" is literally true. I have seen the power of positive thinking for years in my medical practice. I always tell my patients that healing the body is much harder if the mind is full of upset, angry, or fearful images. Healing meditations, when practiced on a regular basis, can be a powerful therapeutic tool. If you enjoy this form of meditation, try designing your own with images that make you feel good.

- Lie on your back in a comfortable position. Inhale and exhale slowly and deeply.

- Visualize a beautiful green meadow full of lovely fragrant flowers. In the middle of this meadow is a golden temple. See the temple emanating peace and healing.

- Visualize yourself entering this temple. You are the only person inside. It is still and peaceful. As you stand inside this temple, you feel a healing energy fill every pore of your body with a warm golden light. This energy feels like a healing balm that relaxes you totally. All anxiety dissolves and fades from your mind. You feel totally at ease.

- Open your eyes and continue your deep, slow breathing for another minute.

Exercise 4: Discovering Muscle Tension

This and the following exercise help you get in touch with your areas of muscle tension, and then teach you how to release that tension. This is an important sequence for women with fibroids or endometriosis who suffer from recurrent menstrual cramps, low back pain, or abdominal discomfort. Many of these symptoms are due in part to the chronically tight and tense muscles that can accompany both problems. Tense muscles tend to have decreased blood circulation and oxygenation, and may accumulate an excess of waste products like carbon dioxide and lactic acid.

Interestingly enough, some women with menstrual cramps and pelvic pain carry tension in these areas throughout the month, even when cramps are absent. They tend to tighten the pelvic and lower abdominal muscles in response to work, relationship, and sexual stresses. Usually, this tensing of the pelvic muscles is an unconscious response that develops over many years and sets up the emotional patterning that triggers cramps. For example, when a woman has uncomfortable feelings about sex or a particular sexual partner, she may tighten these muscles when engaging in or even thinking about sex. Tense muscles also affect a woman's moods, making her more "uptight" and irritable.

Muscular and emotional tension usually coexist. Movement is

one effective way of breaking up these habitual patterns of muscle holding and contracting. When muscles are loose and limber, a woman tends to feel more relaxed and in a better mood. Anxiety tends to fade away, replaced by a sense of expansiveness and calm.

- Lie in a comfortable position. Allow your arms to rest comfortably by your sides, palms down, on the surface next to you.

- Now, raise just the right hand and arm and hold it elevated for 15 seconds.

- Notice if your forearm feels tight and tense or if the muscles are soft and pliable.

- Now, let your hand and arm drop down and relax. The arm muscles will relax too.

- As you lie still, notice any other parts of your body that feel tense, any muscles that feel tight and sore. You may notice a constant dull aching in certain muscles. Tense muscles block blood flow and cut off the supply of nutrients to the tissues. In response to the poor oxygenation, the muscle produces lactic acid, which further increases muscular discomfort.

Exercise 5: Progressive Muscle Relaxation

- Lie in a comfortable position. Allow your arms to rest at your sides, palms down, on the surface next to you.

- Inhale and exhale slowly and deeply.

- Clench your hands into fists and hold them tightly for 15 seconds. As you do this, relax the rest of your body. Visualize the tense part contracting, becoming tighter and tighter.

- Then let your hands relax. On relaxing, see a golden light flowing into the entire body, making all your muscles soft and pliable.

- Now, tense and relax the following parts of your body in this order: face, shoulders, back, stomach, pelvis, legs, feet, and toes. Hold each part tensed for 15 seconds and then relax your body for 30 seconds before going on to the next part.

- Finish the exercise by shaking your hands and imagining the remaining tension flowing out of your fingertips.

Exercise 6: Affirmations

Affirmations are positive statements that describe how you want your body to be. They are very important because they align your mind with your body in a positive way. As the healing meditations (exercise 3) achieve this goal through the use of positive images, affirmations do it through the power of suggestion. Your state of health is determined in part by the interaction between your mind and body via the thousands of messages you send yourself each day with your thoughts. You can aggravate your fibroid and endometrial menstrual bleeding and cramps as well as pelvic discomfort with negative thoughts, because when your body believes it is sick, it behaves accordingly. Thus, it is essential to cultivate a positive belief system and a positive body image as part of your healing program. It is not enough to follow an excellent diet and a vigorous exercise routine when you are in the process of healing menstrual cramps. You must also tell your body that it is a well, fully functional system. I have seen people stay ill and sabotage their healing program by sending themselves a barrage of negative messages.

Sit in a comfortable position. Repeat the following affirmations. Repeat three times those that are particularly important to you.

- My female system is strong and healthy.

- My hormonal levels are perfectly balanced and regulated.

- My body chemistry is healthy and balanced.

- I go through my monthly menstrual cycle with ease and comfort.

- My menstrual flow self-regulates. I have light to moderate bleeding.

- My body is relaxed and pain-free.
- My vaginal muscles are relaxed and comfortable.
- My cervix and uterus are relaxed and pain-free.
- My uterus is normal in size and shape.
- My menstrual flow leaves my body easily and effortlessly each month.
- My body feels wonderful as I start each monthly period.
- I barely know that my body is getting ready to menstruate.
- I feel wonderful each month before I menstruate.
- My uterus is relaxed and receptive; I welcome my monthly period.
- My low back muscles feel supple and pliable with each menstrual cycle.
- I am relaxed and at ease as my period approaches.
- I desire a well-balanced and healthful diet.
- I eat only the foods that are good for my female body.
- It is a real pleasure to take good care of my body.
- I do the level of exercise that keeps my body healthy and supple.
- I handle stress easily and in a relaxed manner.
- I love my body; I feel at ease in my body.
- My body is pain-free and relaxed.

Exercise 7: Visualizations

Visualization exercises help you lay down the mental blueprint for a healthier body. This powerful technique can stimulate positive chemical and hormonal changes in your body to help create the desired outcome. Through positive visualization, you are imaging your body the way you want it to function and be. The body can modify its chemical and hormonal output in response to this technique and move toward a state of improved health. As a result, you may find this technique useful for reducing the symptoms and severity of both fibroids and endometriosis.

Patients with many types of illnesses have used visualization to great benefit. The technique was pioneered by Carl Simonton, M.D., a cancer radiation therapist who used visualization with his patients. Aware that his patients tended to see their cancer as a "big destructive monster," he had them instead visualize their immune systems as big white knights or white sharks attacking the small and insignificant cancer cells and destroying them (instead of the other way around). In many cases, he saw his patients' health improve.

This visualization exercise for fibroids and endometriosis uses an "erasure" image that helps you see your fibroids or the endometrial implants melt away and disappear. Simply skip the part of the exercise that does not pertain to your symptoms.

- Sit in a comfortable position.

- Close your eyes. Begin to breathe deeply. Inhale and let the air out slowly. Feel your body begin to relax.

- Imagine that you can look, as if through a magic mirror, deep inside your own body.

- Focus on any areas of your reproductive tract that you sense contain endometrial implants. See any lesions, cysts, or scarring that the endometriosis has caused. You may visualize the actual implants, or you may simply see the endometriosis as discolored areas within your body (colors such as gray or brown are common).

- Next, imagine a large eraser, like the kind used to erase chalk marks, coming into your pelvic area. See this eraser rubbing the areas of endometriosis. See these implants begin to loosen, shrink, and finally disappear.

- Now, look at your female organs. See your uterus and ovaries. They are an attractive pink color. Your uterus is relaxed and supple. Any fibroid tumors are melting away as you look at them. Your uterus is becoming its normal size and shape. Your uterus has good blood circulation. Look at your ovaries. They are extremely healthy and put out just the right levels of hormones. They are shiny and pink and look like two almonds. The fallopian tubes that pick up the eggs and bring them to the uterus are totally open and healthy.

- Look at your abdominal and low back muscles. They are soft and pliable with a healthy muscle tone. They are relaxed and free of tension during your menstrual period. Your abdomen is flat and your fluid balance is perfect in your pelvic area.

- Look at your entire body and enjoy the sense of peace and calm running through your body. You feel wonderful.

- Stop visualizing the scene, and focus on your deep breathing, inhaling and exhaling slowly.

- You open your eyes and feel very good. Visualizing this scene should take a minute or two. Linger on any images that particularly please you.

More Stress-Reduction Techniques

The rest of this chapter explains other techniques that I have found useful for relaxing tight and tense muscles. You can also use these methods to induce deep emotional relaxation. Try them for a delightful experience.

Hydrotherapy

For centuries, people have used warm water to relax their muscles and calm their mood. You can create your own "spa" at home by adding relaxing ingredients to the bath water. I have found two recipes extremely useful in relieving muscle pain and tension related to fibroids or endometriosis.

Recipe 1: Alkaline Bath. Run a tub of warm water. Heat will increase your menstrual flow, so keep the water a little cooler if that is a problem. Add one cup of sea salt and one cup of bicarbonate of soda to the tub. As this is a highly alkaline mixture, I recommend using it only once or twice a month. I've found it very helpful in reducing cramps and calming anxiety and irritability. Soak for 20 minutes. You will probably feel relaxed and sleepy after this bath. Try it at night before going to sleep. You will probably wake up feeling refreshed and energized the following day. Heat of any kind helps to release muscle tension. You may also want to try a hot water bottle or a heating pad to relieve cramps.

Recipe 2: Hydrogen Peroxide Bath. This is one of my personal favorites. Hydrogen peroxide is a combination of water and oxygen. By adding it to your bath, you "hyperoxygenate" the water. This helps to induce muscle relaxation. Hydrogen peroxide is inexpensive and can be purchased from your local drug store or supermarket. I usually add three pint bottles of the 3-percent solution to a full tub of warm water and soak for up to 30 minutes. If you use the stronger food- or technical-grade hydrogen peroxide (35-percent strength), add only 6 ounces. With the more concentrated peroxide, be sure to avoid direct contact with your hands or eyes and keep it stored in a cool place, as it is a very powerful oxidizer.

Sound

Music can have a tremendously relaxing effect on our minds and bodies. For women with fibroid- or endometriosis-related cramps and pain, I recommend slow, quiet music—classical music is particularly good. This type of music can have a pronounced beneficial effect on your physiological functions. It can slow your pulse and heart rate, lower your blood pressure, and decrease your levels of stress hormones. It can also help reduce anxiety and induce sleep for women with cramps. Equally beneficial are nature sounds, such as ocean waves and rainfall; these sounds can also induce a sense of peace and relaxation. I have patients who keep tapes of nature sounds in their car and at home for use when they feel stressed. Play relaxing music often as your menstrual cycle approaches and you are aware of increased levels of emotional and physical tension.

Biofeedback Therapy

Biofeedback therapy is an effective way to relieve pain of all kinds caused by muscular tension, as well as poor circulation caused by narrowing of the blood-vessel diameter. Constriction of the skeletal muscles and the smooth muscle of the blood-vessel wall usually occurs on an unconscious basis, so a person is not even aware that it's happening. A variety of factors, including emotional stress and nutritional or chemical imbalances, can trigger this involuntary muscle tension. This constriction can worsen problems such as fibroids, endometriosis, migraine headaches, and high blood pressure.

Using biofeedback therapy, people learn to recognize when they are tensing their muscles. Once this response is understood, fibroid and endometriosis sufferers can learn to relax their muscles to help relieve the pain. Since muscle relaxation both decreases muscular discomfort and improves blood flow, either factor can be monitored. For relief of cramps, women can learn how to implement biofeedback therapy through a series of training sessions, requiring about 10 to 15 thirty-minute office visits with a trained professional. During these sessions, a thermometer is inserted into the vagina like a tampon. The thermometer is connected to a digital readout machine that monitors the woman's internal temperature. The professional teaches her how to consciously change her vaginal temperature. Even a slight rise in the temperature indicates better blood flow and muscle relaxation in the pelvic area, with a concomitant relief of menstrual pain.

After the training sessions, most women are able to raise their temperature at will and thereby control their own cramps. I went through biofeedback training many years ago and found that it had a significant effect on my level of muscle tension. Many hospitals and university centers have biofeedback units, as do stress management clinics, so it is relatively easy to find a treatment facility that offers this type of therapy.

Putting Your Stress-Reduction Program Together

This chapter has introduced many different ways to reset your mind and body to help make menstruation a calm and relaxed time of the month and ease the symptoms of fibroids and endometriosis. Try each exercise at least once. Experiment with them until you find the combination that works for you. Doing all seven exercises will take no longer than 20 to 30 minutes, depending on how much time you wish to spend with each one. Ideally, you should do the exercises at least a few minutes each day. Over time, they will help you gain insight into your negative beliefs and change them into positive new ones. Your ability to cope with stress should improve tremendously.

Suggested Reading

Benson, R., and M. Klipper. *Relaxation Response*. New York: Avon, 1976.

Brennan, B. A. *Hands of Light*. New York: Bantam, 1987.

Davis, M. M., M. Eshelman, and E. Eshelman. *The Relaxation and Stress Reduction Workbook*. Oakland, CA: New Harbinger Publications, 1982.

Gawain, S. *Creative Visualization*. San Rafael, CA: New World Publishing, 1978.

Gawain, S. *Living in the Light*. Mill Valley, CA: Whatever Publishing, 1986.

Kripalu Center for Holistic Health. *The Self-Health Guide*. Lenox, MA: Kripalu Publications, 1980.

Loehr, J., and J. Migdow. *Take a Deep Breath*. New York: Villard Books, 1986.

Miller, E. *Self-Imagery*. Berkeley, CA: Celestial Arts, 1986.

Ornstein, R., and D. Sobel. *Healthy Pleasures*. Reading, MA: Addison-Wesley, 1989.

8

Breathing Exercises

$\mathcal{B}$reathing exercises are a simple yet powerful way to reduce fibroid- and endometriosis-related pain and cramps. Through therapeutic breathing, you can relax and loosen your muscles, decrease sensations of pain, lower your anxiety level, and generate a feeling of internal peace and calm. This process grants you a degree of voluntary control over your discomfort. Many of my patients find the combination of breathing exercises and stress-reduction techniques to be very empowering.

When you are breathing slowly and deeply, you take large amounts of oxygen into your circulatory system, where it binds to the red blood cells as it travels through the arteries and veins. Oxygen enables the cells to produce and utilize energy, and to remove waste products through the production of carbon dioxide. These waste products are cleared through exhalation by the lungs. Thus, the whole body needs optimal levels of oxygen for its normal cycle of building, repair, and elimination. Although there are no specific studies on the use of breathing exercises in patients with fibroids and endometriosis, I believe that the stress-reducing benefits may help your body limit and repair the damage caused by endometriosis, as well as normalize hormonal output and thereby limit the growth of fibroids.

When you are in physical and emotional distress, oxygen levels decrease. Breathing tends to become jagged, erratic, and shallow. You may find yourself breathing too fast or with severe pain. You may stop breathing altogether and hold your breath for prolonged periods of time without even realizing it. None of these breathing patterns is healthful. Anxious breathing is often linked to other unhealthy physiological reactions that reflect your body's state of stress. When you have cramps and pain, besides lowering the oxygen level in your body, you tend to tighten your muscles, constrict blood flow, elevate your pulse rate and heartbeat, and stimulate the output of stressful chemicals from your glands in response to the pelvic discomfort. Waste products like carbon dioxide and lactic acid also accumulate in your muscles and other tissues.

Therapeutic breathing exercises provide a way to break up this pattern and help the body return to equilibrium. It is important to do the breathing exercises in a slow and regular manner. First, find a comfortable position. Some exercises you should do lying on your back; for other exercises, you'll sit up, uncross your arms and legs, and keep your back straight.

Exercise 1: Deep Abdominal Breathing

Deep, slow abdominal breathing is an important technique for the relief of fibroid- and endometriosis-related cramps and pain. It brings adequate oxygen, the fuel for metabolic activity, to all the tissues of your body. Rapid, shallow breathing decreases your oxygen supply and keeps you devitalized. Deep breathing helps relax the entire body and strengthens the muscles in the chest and abdomen. It also helps calm many other physiological processes, such as the rapid pulse rate and heartbeat that often accompany menstrual cramps.

- Lie flat on your back with your knees pulled up. Keep your feet slightly apart. Try to breathe in and out through your nose.

- Inhale deeply. As you breathe in, allow your stomach to relax so that the air flows into your abdomen. Your stomach should balloon out as you breathe in. Visualize your lungs filling up with air so that your chest swells out.

- Imagine that the air you breathe is filling your body with energy.

- Exhale deeply. As you breathe out, let your stomach and chest collapse. Imagine the air being pushed out, first from your abdomen and then from your lungs.

Exercise 2: Peaceful, Slow Breathing

Breathing slowly and peacefully can actually decrease anxiety and help promote a sense of inner calm and quiet. Such breathing helps our mind to slow down and our emotions be happier and more harmonious. Life feels good. When we are calm, we make better decisions and relate to those around us in a healthier way. Breathing slowly can also calm our physical responses by helping to balance autonomic nervous system function. The autonomic nervous system regulates functions that we're usually not aware of, such as circulation of the blood, muscle tension, pulse rate, breathing, and glandular function. The autonomic nervous system is divided into two parts that oppose and complement each other, the sympathetic and parasympathetic systems. The sympathetic nervous system is linked to tension and the "fight-or-flight" response of fear and panic, while the parasympathetic nervous system regulates body responses that are relaxed and calm. When women have menstrual cramps and low back pain, the sympathetic nervous system is in overdrive. The pain sensation causes muscles to tense. Furthermore, the pulse rate tends to accelerate and the blood vessels to constrict. Slow, peaceful breathing is a way to calm down these stress responses and bring the body back to a state of balance. By slowing down our breathing, we slow down our other physiologic responses. Our muscles relax and our blood vessels dilate; we have restored a state of equilibrium.

- Lie flat on your back with your knees pulled up. Keep your feet slightly apart. Try to breathe in and out through your nose.

- Inhale deeply. As you breathe in, allow your stomach to relax so that the air flows into your abdomen. Let your stomach balloon out as you breathe in. Visualize the lowest parts of your lungs filling up with air.

- Imagine that the air you are breathing in is filled with peace and calm. A sensation of peace and calm is filling every cell of your body. Your whole body feels warm and relaxed as you breathe in this air. Now, exhale deeply. As you breathe out, imagine the air being pushed out from the bottom of your lungs to the top.

- Repeat this sequence until your entire body feels relaxed and your breathing is slow and regular.

Exercise 3: Grounding Breath

Women in pain and discomfort often lose a sense of being grounded, or rooted to the earth. Some women report a sensation of numbness in their legs and feet. They may say they feel as if they have no legs at all. This is due in part to the fact that fibroid- and endometriosis-related pelvic cramps and low back pain cause leg muscles to tighten and blood circulation and oxygenation to the lower extremities to decrease. Thus the women lose a sense of owning their legs. When a person is physically ungrounded, functioning mentally becomes difficult, so these women have a hard time focusing and concentrating. When your body is uncomfortable, you may have difficulty sitting at a desk and working through your projects for the day in a coherent manner. This breathing exercise will help you to ground and focus both physically and mentally. You should feel much more stable and focused by the end of this exercise.

- Sit upright in a chair. Be sure you are in a comfortable position. Keep your feet slightly apart. Try to breathe in and out through your nose.

- Inhale deeply. As you breathe in, allow your stomach to relax so that the air flows into your abdomen. Let your stomach balloon out as you breathe in. Visualize the lowest parts of your lungs filling up with air. Hold your inhalation.

- See a large, thick cord running from the bottom of your buttocks to the center of the earth. Follow the cord all the way down and see it fasten securely to the earth's center. Run two smaller cords from the bottom of your feet down to the center of the earth also.

- As you exhale, gently push your buttocks into the rest of your chair. Become aware of your buttocks, thighs, calves, ankles, and feet. Feel their strength and solidity.

- Repeat this exercise several times until you feel fully present and grounded.

Exercise 4: Muscle-Tension Release Breathing

This exercise will help you get in touch with and release general muscle tension and tightness. Often when the uterus, abdominal muscles, and low back are tight, you unconsciously tense up muscles throughout your entire body, making the neck, shoulders, and other vulnerable areas tense, too. You can have tense muscles in other parts of the body without being aware of it. This exercise will help you focus on any tension that you are carrying in your upper body. It will also help you take your focus off your cramps. As you relax and release the muscles in your neck and shoulders, you will also release muscle tension in your entire body. This is a good exercise to do while walking, engaging in sports, or taking care of desk work, to get in touch with any muscle tension you may be carrying.

- Sit upright in a chair. (If you perform this exercise while walking or involved in another activity, just be in a position that is as comfortable as possible.) Be sure you are in a comfortable position. Keep your feet slightly apart. Try to breathe in and out through your nose.

- Inhale and exhale deeply. As you breathe, let your head move from side to side. Keep your shoulders down and try to touch your ear to your shoulder. As you do this movement, imagine that your neck is made out of putty, allowing your head to move in a supple, relaxed movement from left to right.

- Now inhale and pull your shoulders up toward your ears. Hold your breath and keep your shoulders in a hunched position. Exhale and let your shoulders drop back into a relaxed, comfortable position. Repeat this several times.

- Inhale and exhale deeply as you roll your shoulders forward. Make a large, slow, circular motion with your shoulders. Then, roll your shoulders back slowly. Repeat this several times.

- Inhale and exhale deeply, keeping the rest of your body still and relaxed. Repeat this several times.

Exercise 5: Emotional Cleansing Breath

During my years of medical practice, I have seen menstrual cramps, inflammatory pain, and even menstrual bleeding problems intensify when women are under emotional stress. The more day-to-day stress you have over family, work, and other personal issues, the more this can aggravate your fibroids and endometriosis. In fact, many of my patients have told me they believe that their unhealed personal relationships, as well as sexual problems, are significant emotional triggers for their cramps and pain.

This particular exercise uses breathing to help you release any negative feelings, chronic anger, or upset that you may be harboring. The more time you spend cleansing old negative emotional patterns, the less impact these feelings can have on your sensitive female reproductive tract with the onset of each menstruation.

- Lie flat on your back with your knees pulled up. Keep your feet slightly apart. Try to breathe in and out through your nose.

- Inhale deeply and see yourself enveloped in a soft white light. Breathe this light into every cell of your body. This is a cleansing light and can help wash away fear, anger, anxiety, and other negative feelings.

- As you exhale deeply, feel the light washing these emotions away.

- Repeat this exercise until you feel emotionally peaceful and clear.

Exercise 6: Color Breathing with Red and Blue

Color breathing (exercises 6 and 7) has been used in more than one ancient tradition to heal the body and strengthen the body's energy field. Intuitives in our culture can see this energy field as light or colors emanating from the body. When a person is calm, relaxed, and healthy, the energy field looks radiant and full of colors. The colors are bright and harmonious, and each one corresponds to specific parts of the body.

When we are feeling pain or tension, as often happens with the chronic symptoms of fibroids or endometriosis, we literally lose light and color. Our energy field looks more discordant and jagged, and the colors become duller, or muddied. Color breathing is a technique that can help strengthen and heal the energy field as well as the body itself. As you breathe in the healing colors, the parts of your body that are in pain and discomfort often begin to relax and feel healthier again. Tension and cramping is replaced by a sensation of lightness and peace.

- Sit or lie in a comfortable position. Take a deep breath and visualize that the earth below you is a deep scarlet red. This color extends 50 feet below you into the earth. Imagine that you are opening up energy centers on the bottoms of your feet. As you inhale, visualize the deep scarlet red color filling up your feet. Draw this color up your legs and into your pelvic area. See it first filling up your legs, then your lower back, and finally your pelvis. Your uterus is filling with a beautiful deep scarlet red color. As you exhale, see this color dissolving and washing away any areas of fibroids or endometriosis in your body. See this color flow out of your uterus and lower back and fill the air around you. Exhale the deep scarlet red slowly out of your lungs. Repeat this process 5 times.

- Visualize that the earth beneath you is a dark, inky indigo blue. As you inhale, draw this color into the bottoms of your feet. Let the color fill your legs, lower back, and pelvic region. Then see this indigo blue fill your uterus. As you exhale, see this color dissolving and washing away any areas of fibroids or endometriosis in your body. See this color flow out of your uterus and lower back and fill the air around you. Exhale the deep indigo blue slowly out of your lungs. Repeat this process 5 times.

Exercise 7: Color Breathing with Golden Light

- Sit or lie in a comfortable position.

- Imagine a cloud of beautiful golden energy surrounding you. As you take a deep breath, inhale the golden energy and visualize it flowing through your body and into your uterus, pelvic area, and lower back. This is a healing energy—it warms and relaxes your uterus, lower abdominal muscles, and lower back.

- Hold the inhalation as long as it is comfortable. Let this golden cloud pick up all your pain and tension.

- Then, exhale this energy out through your lungs and let it be carried away from you.

- Repeat this process as many times as needed until the pain is replaced by a feeling of peace and calm.

9

Physical Exercise

$\mathcal{E}$xercise is an important part of a fibroid- and endometriosis-relief program because of its role in pain relief and the prevention of the menstrual pain and cramps that accompany these conditions. To better understand how exercise can provide relief, let us look first at the physiological effects that fibroids and endometriosis produce in your body. Many women with both conditions complain of pain and discomfort. This includes pain at midcycle, in the two weeks prior to the onset of menstruation, with sexual intercourse, and even with bowel movements and urination if the endometrial implants have invaded the neighboring organs. With fibroids, these symptoms are often due to direct pressure from the fibroids on other pelvic organs. Endometriosis causes internal bleeding in the pelvis which worsens inflammation. Endometrial implants can impinge on nerves and neighboring organ systems and can cause inflammation and scarring in the pelvic tissues.

In response to the discomfort caused by these two conditions, women often involuntarily contract the muscles of the pelvis, low back, and uterus. This is a natural response to pain. Tight and tense uterine and back muscles have decreased blood flow and oxygenation. Waste products such as excessive carbon dioxide can accumulate in this physical environment and further worsen symptoms. In addition, the pain of menstrual cramps causes breathing to become rapid and shallow. Less oxygen is taken in through respiration, which further decreases the oxygen available to the pelvic region. Metabolism of the muscles becomes less efficient, and fluid retention can become a problem in the pelvic area as well as the ankles and feet. Many women complain of drawing pains in their thighs and aching sensations in their legs.

Aerobic exercise helps to relieve these symptoms. Playing tennis, walking, swimming, and dancing require deep breathing and active movement. With better respiration, oxygenation and blood flow to the pelvic area improve. The vigorous pumping action of the muscles that occurs with these activities helps reduce the congestive symptoms of menstrual cramps by moving blood and other fluids from the pelvic region. Exercise of this type should not, however, be done too vigorously. "Going for the burn" is not a good idea for women with endometriosis. Muscle fatigue from overexercise causes muscles to become oxygen-deficient and use up their reserve energy stores. This can intensify the pain symptoms of fibroids and endometriosis.

Exercise also produces significant psychological benefits to sufferers of fibroids and endometriosis. Improved oxygenation and blood flow benefit the brain as well as the pelvic muscles. For optimal functioning, the brain demands a healthy share of the body's available nutrients. When the brain and nervous systems are functioning well, exercise triggers an increased output of endorphins. These chemicals made by the brain have a natural opiate effect. Endorphins are thought to produce the "runner's high" that marathoners experience. Many women patients tell me that moderate and relaxed exercise is their most effective form of stress management, and that exercise produces a sense of peace and tranquillity unmatched by anything else they do.

Another way aerobic exercise might help to reduce anxiety and calm the mood is by helping balance the autonomic nervous system. The autonomic nervous system regulates the "fight-or-flight" response that many women experience around the time of their menstrual period. When this system is in overdrive, small life worries can become magnified out of proportion because the body reacts to these small stresses as if they were life-threatening issues. Regular exercise helps lessen the intensity of this response. This can be a real benefit for fibroid and endometriosis sufferers, many of whom lead complex and demanding lives.

I also recommend that women with fibroid- and endometriosis-related menstrual cramps and low back pain consider doing flexibility and stretching exercises as part of their physical activity program. These exercises help prevent cramps and low back pain by strengthening the back and abdominal muscles. By balancing muscle tension through controlled, slow movement, stretching can also help to improve posture. When done properly, stretching exercises bring an awareness of how the parts of the body are aligned spatially with respect to each other.

In summary, exercise brings many healthful benefits to women who suffer from the symptoms of fibroids and endometriosis. I recommend that women with these problems follow a regular program of physical activity for cramps throughout the entire month. Though exercise does not cure fibroids and endometriosis, it can help alleviate both the physical and emotional symptoms that accompany these conditions. The remainder of this chapter describes a sequence of stretches and exercises useful in the relief of menstrual distress.

General Fitness and Flexibility Exercises

As part of your self-help program, the following set of exercises are good for mobility, flexibility, and relaxation. You can use them with great benefit during the premenstrual and menstrual time of the month to help loosen the joints in your lower body and decrease muscle stiffness and tension. You can also do these exercises throughout the month. Practiced on a regular basis, they will improve your vigor and energy level. The same exercises can help warm up tense and tight muscles before you engage in sports or athletic events.

I do many of these exercises myself and have found them to be very helpful during times of physical and emotional stress and tension. They have helped me tremendously to stay loose and flexible.

The following guidelines will help you perform the exercises safely and efficiently, without undue stress.

- During the first week or two of your program, try all these exercises. Then put together your own routine based on the exercises that provide the most benefit. You may find that you want to use all of them on a regular basis or perhaps only a few of them. Warm-ups should always precede any sports or athletic event.

- Perform the exercises in a relaxed and unhurried manner. Be sure to set aside adequate time—about 30 minutes—so you do not feel rushed. Your work area should be quiet, peaceful, and uncluttered.

- Wear loose, comfortable clothing. It is better to exercise without socks to give your feet complete freedom of movement and to prevent slipping.

- Evacuate your bowels or bladder before you begin the exercises. Wait at least two hours after eating to exercise.

- Choose a flat area and work on a mat or a blanket. This will make you more comfortable while you do the exercises.

- When beginning an exercise, pay close attention to the initial instructions. Look at the placement of the body as shown in the photographs. This is very important, for you are much more likely to have relief of your symptoms if you do the exercise properly.

- Try to visualize the exercise in your mind, then follow with proper placement of the body.

- Move slowly through the exercise. This helps promote flexibility of the muscles and prevent injury.

- Always rest for a few minutes after doing the exercises.

- Try to practice these movements on a regular basis. A short session every day is best. If that is not possible, then try to practice them every other day.

Exercise 1: Deep Breathing

Deep, slow abdominal breathing is essential for women with fibroids and endometriosis. It expands your lungs and allows you to bring adequate oxygen, the fuel for metabolic activity, to all the tissues of your body. Deep breathing will relax tight and contracted pelvic, abdominal, and low back muscles, thereby helping to relieve menstrual pain and distress. It also helps to relax the entire body and strengthens the muscles in the chest and abdomen. Deep breathing helps to stabilize mood and reduce both depression and anxiety, so it is very important for emotional well-being. In contrast, rapid, shallow breathing decreases your oxygen supply, which builds up lactic acid in the pelvic muscles, keeping them tense and tight.

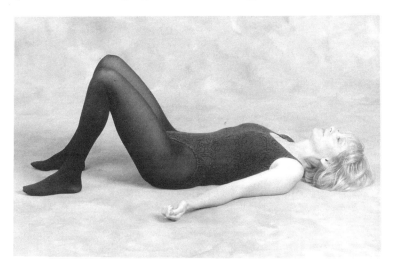

- Lie flat on your back with your knees pulled up. Keep your feet slightly apart. Try to breathe in and out through your nose.

- Inhale deeply. As you breathe in, allow your stomach to relax so that the air flows into your abdomen. Your stomach should balloon out as you breathe in. Visualize your lungs filling up with air so that your chest swells out.

- Imagine that the air you breathe is filling your body with energy.

- Exhale deeply. As you breathe out, let your stomach and chest collapse. Imagine the air being pushed out, first from your abdomen and then from your lungs.

Exercise 2: Total Body Muscle Relaxation

Women with fibroids and endometriosis frequently have muscle groups that are tense and tight because of inadequate oxygenation and blood flow. Lactic acid tends to accumulate in these muscles, and muscle tension can become a chronic problem. This is particularly true during midcycle, at ovulation, and during the two weeks preceding menstruation. Shifts in the body's hormonal and mineral balance predispose women with these problems toward muscle tension. Also, the muscles in the pelvic region may tense in response to the internal bleeding, inflammation, and other internal changes caused by the endometriosis itself. Regular physical activity effectively breaks up this pattern of chronically tight muscles. During the second half of the menstrual cycle, it is very important to keep the muscles loose and flexible. Besides feeling more relaxed, supple muscles have a beneficial effect on the mood and induce an overall sense of peace and calm. The following exercise helps you to get in touch with the parts of your body that feel tense and contracted. It will also aid you in releasing muscle tension.

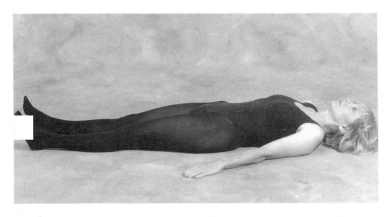

- Lie in a comfortable position. Allow your arms to rest limply, palms down, on the surface next to you. Breathe slowly and deeply as you do this exercise.

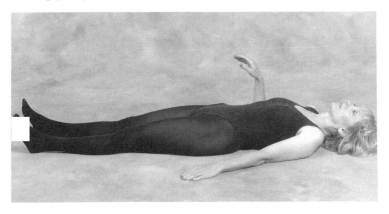

- Raise your right hand off the floor and hold it there for 15 seconds. Notice any tension in your forearm or upper arm. Let your hand slowly relax and rest on the floor. The hand and arm muscles should relax. As you lie there, notice any other parts of your body where you are carrying tension.

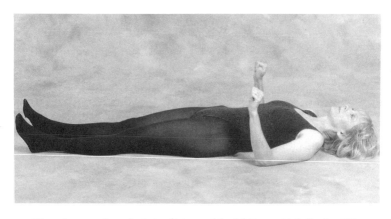

- Clench your hands into fists and hold them tightly for 15 seconds. As you do this, relax the rest of your body. Then let your hands relax.

- Now, tense and relax the following parts of your body in this order: face, shoulders, back, stomach, pelvis, legs, feet, and toes. Hold each part tensed for 15 seconds and then relax your body for 30 seconds before going on to the next part.

- Visualize the tense part contracting, becoming tighter and tighter. On relaxing, see the energy flowing into the entire body like a gentle wave, making all the muscles soft and pliable.

- Finish the exercise by shaking your hands. Imagine the remaining tension flowing out of your fingertips.

Exercise 3: Energizing Sequence

The pain and blood loss that accompany fibroids and endometriosis can leave women feeling tired and depleted for several days to two weeks per month. This exercise sequence increases your energy, releases muscle tension, and improves circulation. The exercise stimulates movement and energy flow through all muscles of the body, starting from the legs and moving up to the top of the head. In traditional Indian healing models, these exercises are thought to stimulate the seven *chakras* or vital energy centers of the body. This sequence emphasizes the muscles of the lower extremities, low back, pelvis, and abdomen, since they are particularly affected by fibroids and endometriosis.

Do the steps in this sequence slowly, so as not to stress the body. You will feel the benefits this exercise can have on your energy level if you don't rush through the steps or do them too hard. As your strength and flexibility improve, you may want to do the steps a little more vigorously.

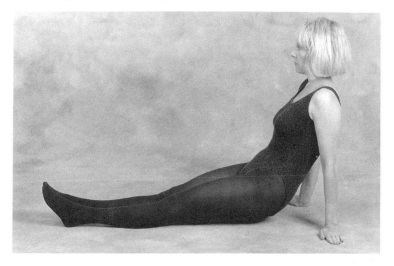

Legs and Hips

- Sit on the floor with your legs stretched straight in front of you. Place your hands on the floor behind you. Lift your buttocks off the floor and bounce gently on the base of your spine.

- Repeat 5 times.

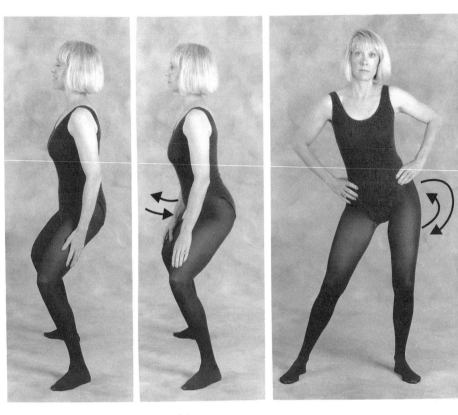

Legs and Pelvis

- Stand with your legs spread apart about 2 feet. Point your feet out at a comfortable angle.

- Rock your pelvis back and forth.

- Repeat 10 times. Then rotate your hips in a circular fashion, first moving them clockwise and then counterclockwise.

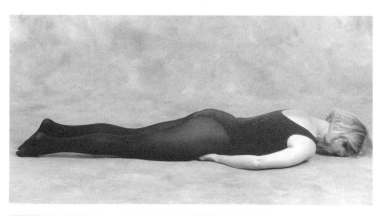

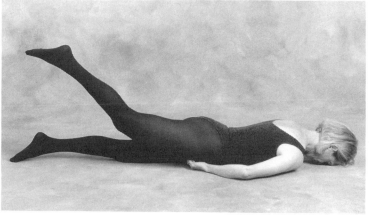

Pelvis and Lower Abdomen

- Lie on your stomach, placing your fists under your hips. Rest your forehead on the floor.

- As you inhale, raise your right leg with an upward thrust, keeping your hips on your fists. Hold for 5 to 20 seconds if possible.

- Lower the leg and slowly bring it back to the original position.

- Repeat several times. Then do the exercise on the left side.

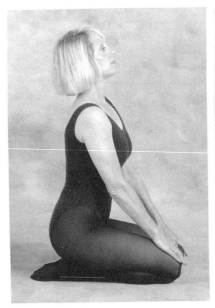
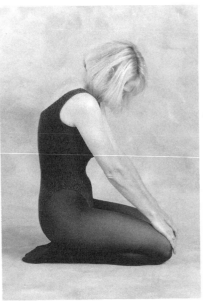

Abdomen and Chest

- Sit on your heels with your hands placed on your knees. As you inhale, arch your back and stretch to expand your chest up and out.

- As you exhale, slump down to curve your back.

- Repeat several times.

Exercise 4: Lower Back Arch

This exercise helps loosen the lower back muscles and improves flexibility of the spine. It can also combat tiredness in women who experience deceased energy during the onset of menstruation.

- Stand with your legs spread 1 foot apart. Point your feet straight ahead.

Place your hands around your waist with your thumbs pressing into your lower back.

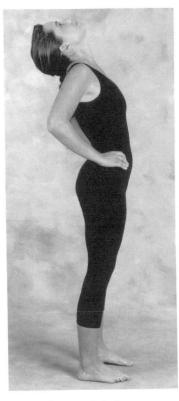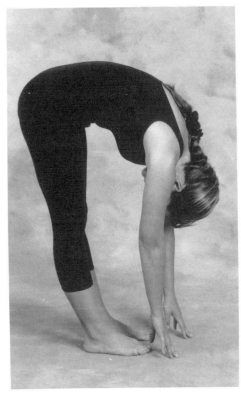

As you inhale, curve your back into an arch with your head held back.

- As you exhale, let the weight of your body bend you forward and curve in an arch, so that your head almost touches your knees. Hold this position for a few seconds.

Return to the original position as you inhale. Do this exercise slowly and repeat several times.

Exercise 5: Abdominal Muscle Release

This exercise helps to release lower and upper abdominal tension. Many women with endometriosis often have digestive symptoms such as nausea and bowel changes. Fibroids may impinge on the bowel, causing pressure symptoms. This twist exercise helps reduce the tension in the abdominal muscles that can worsen these symptoms.

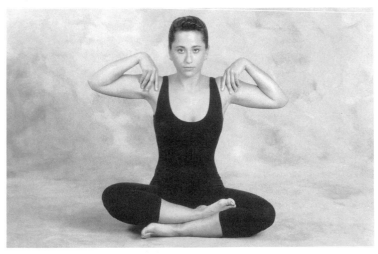

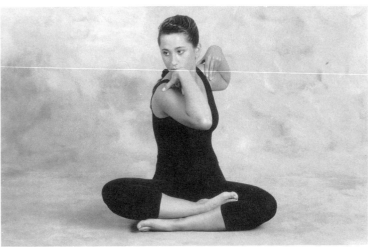

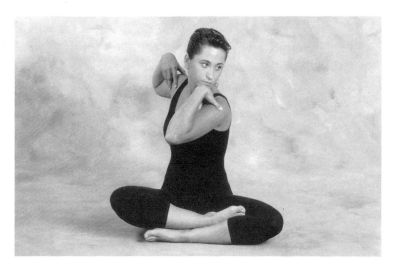

- Sit on the floor with your legs out in front. Place your hands on your shoulders with your fingers in front and your thumbs in back. Be sure to keep your spine straight and inhale deeply.

- As you inhale, twist your head, chest, and abdomen to the left. As you exhale, twist your body to the right.

- Do this exercise 4 times. Then reverse directions and repeat the sequence.

Exercise 6: Lower Back Release

This exercise promotes relaxation, specifically in the lower back, hips, and abdominal muscles. With the alternating tensing and releasing of the abdominal and hip muscles, along with controlled heavy breathing, the entire middle and lower body become looser and more supple. You may also notice a decrease in anxiety and emotional tension after this exercise.

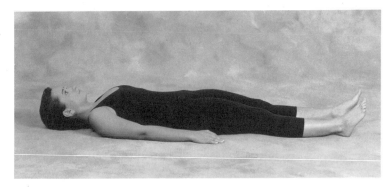

- Lie on your back with your legs together. Raise your feet 6 to 8 inches off the ground; then raise your head and shoulders 6 inches, also.

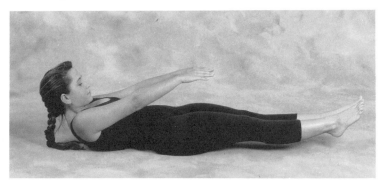

- Point to your toes with your fingertips, keeping your arms straight and your eyes fixed on your toes. Then, breathe through your nose deeply to a count of 20.

- Lower your legs and head and relax.

- Rest for a count of 30.

- Repeat this exercise several times.

Exercise 7: Lower Back Twist

This exercise allows you to twist over to the side, which is actually a natural position for your body to assume when you are feeling pelvic discomfort. This gentle stretch helps to lengthen the muscles in the lower back as well as along the entire spine. It also helps to align the lumbar spine. Many women find that this exercise helps relieve pelvic tension and discomfort.

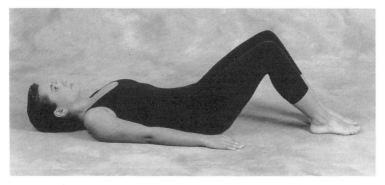

- Lie on your back with your knees bent, feet placed flat on the floor.

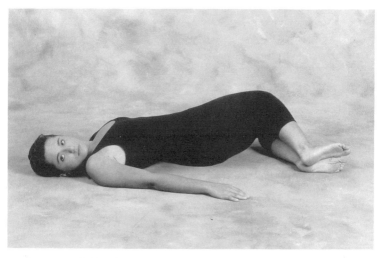

- As you exhale, slowly let your knees and hips fall to the left as you turn your head to the right. Inhale and bring your knees back together to the center.

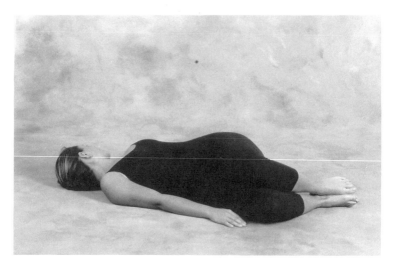

- Then exhale again and reverse direction, letting your knees and hips fall to the right as you turn your head to the left.
- Repeat this exercise slowly several times, alternating sides.

Suggested Reading

Caillet, R., M.D., and L. Gross. *The Rejuvenation Strategy.* New York: Pocket Books, 1987.

Hanna, T. *Somatics.* Reading, MA: Addison-Wesley, 1988.

Huang, C. A. *Tai Ji.* Berkeley, CA: Celestial Arts, 1989.

Jerome, J. *Staying Supple.* New York: Bantam Books, 1987.

Kripalu Center for Holistic Health. *The Self-Health Guide.* Lenox, MA: Kripalu Publications, 1980.

McLish, R., and V. Joyce, Ph.D. *Perfect Parts.* New York: Warner Books, 1987.

Pinkney, C. *Callanetics: 10 Years Younger in 10 Hours.* New York: Avon, 1984.

Solveborn, S. A., M.D. *The Book About Stretching.* New York: Japan Publications, 1985.

Tobias, M., and M. Stewart. *Stretch and Relax.* Tucson, AZ: The Body Press, 1985.

Yoga for Relief of Fibroids & Endometriosis

$\mathcal{T}$he uncomfortable symptoms of fibroids and endometriosis respond well to the gentle stretches of yoga. Yoga exercises that emphasize pelvic movement and flexibility can help treat the menstrual cramps, pelvic congestion, and low back pain that commonly occur with these two problems. Yoga may even help control heavy menstrual flow. The slow, controlled stretching movements that you do in these exercises help relax tense muscles and improve their suppleness and flexibility. They also bring better blood circulation and oxygenation to the tense areas of your lower body, thereby improving the metabolism of the pelvic and back muscles.

Yoga has an additional benefit in that it quiets your moods. The deep breathing and slow movements that characterize these exercises reduce anxiety and irritability and produce a sense of peace—a welcome change for women who have fibroids or endometriosis and also have significant life stress. The stress reduction effects of yoga benefit all body systems, including the reproductive tract and the immune system.

In this chapter I present a series of specific yoga poses that gently stretch every muscle in your body, with specific emphasis on the pelvic and low back region. As well as relieving cramps and discomfort, these exercises energize and balance the female reproductive tract and can help correct underlying hormonal imbalance through improved oxygenation and better circulation to the pelvic area. This can have a beneficial effect on menstrual function. For women who are fatigued from the recurrent menstrual bleeding, pain, and discomfort these conditions cause, yoga can increase vigor and stamina. I do yoga stretches frequently as part of my personal exercise routine.

When doing yoga exercises, it is important that you focus and concentrate on the positions. First, let your mind visualize how the pose is to look, and then follow with the correct body placement for the pose. Pay close attention to the initial instructions. Look at the placement of the body as shown in the photographs. This is very important, for if the pose is practiced properly, you are much more likely to have relief of your symptoms.

Be sure to move slowly through each pose. By taking it slowly, you have greater control over your body movements. You minimize the possibility of injury and maximize the benefit to the particular part of the body affected by the stretch. If you practice these yoga stretches regularly in a slow, unhurried fashion, you will gradually loosen your muscles, ligaments, and joints. You may be surprised at how supple you can become over time.

If you experience any pain or discomfort, you have probably overreached your current ability and should immediately reduce the amount of stretching until you can proceed without discomfort. Be careful, as muscular injuries can take quite a while to heal. If you do strain a muscle, I have found that immediately applying ice to the injured area for 10 minutes is quite helpful. Continue to use the ice pack two to three times a day for several days. If the pain persists, see your doctor.

Follow the breathing instructions provided in the exercises. Most important, do not hold your breath. Allow your breath to flow in and out easily and effortlessly.

Stretch 1: Stretch Pose

This exercise helps stretch and release the low back and pelvic area. Besides relaxing this area and relieving pain, it also helps relieve hemorrhoids and constipation.

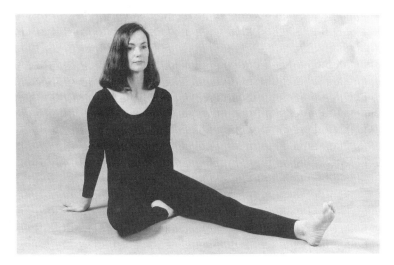

- Sit on the floor with your legs placed straight out in front of you. Bend your right knee and place your right heel in your crotch area. Your left leg remains in a straight position.

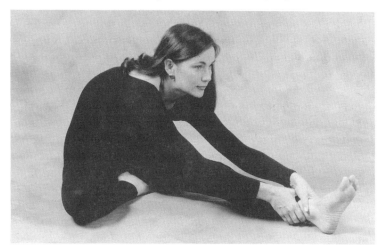

- As you inhale, take hold of your left ankle, straightening your spine. Hold this position for 30 seconds.

- As you exhale, bring your forehead toward your left knee. Hold this position for 30 seconds.

- Repeat this exercise 1 time.

Stretch 2: Pelvic Arch

This is an excellent exercise for stretching the abdominal muscles that are often tightened with menstrual cramps and pain caused by fibroids and endometriosis. It is also helpful in reducing the pelvic congestion that occurs when PMS coexists with these conditions.

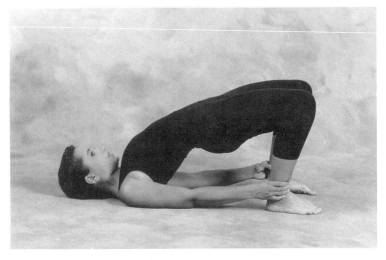

- Lie on your back with your knees bent. Spread your feet apart, flat on the floor.

- Place your hands around your ankles, holding them firmly.

- As you inhale, arch your pelvis up and hold for a few seconds. As you exhale, relax and lower your pelvis.

- Repeat this exercise several times.

Stretch 3: The Locust

This exercise strengthens the lower back, abdomen, buttocks, and legs, and relieves low back pain and menstrual cramps. It also energizes the entire female reproductive tract. Regular practice of this exercise helps improve posture and elimination and will tighten and firm the thighs and hips.

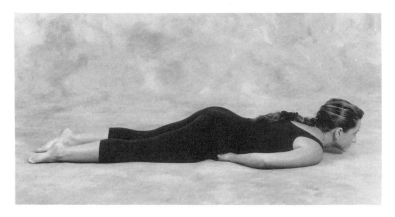

- Lie face down on the floor. Make fists with both your hands and place them under your hips. This prevents compression of the lumbar spine while doing the exercise.

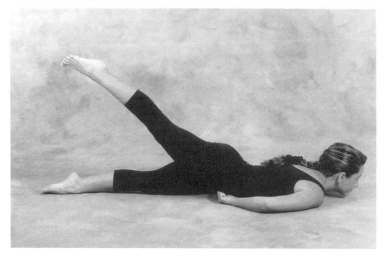

- Straighten your body and raise your right leg with a slow upward thrust as high as you can, keeping your hips on your fists. Hold for 5 to 20 seconds if possible.

- Lower the leg and slowly return to your original position. Repeat with the left leg, then with both legs together. Remember to keep your hips resting on your fists. Repeat 10 times.

Stretch 4: The Bow

This exercise stretches the entire spine and helps relieve low back pain and menstrual cramps due to fibroids and endometriosis. It stretches the abdominal muscles and strengthens the back, hips, and thighs. It also stimulates the digestive organs and endocrine glands. Regular practice of this posture can relieve depression and fatigue by improving your energy and elevating your mood.

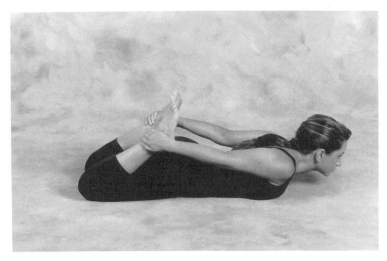

* Lie face down on the floor, arms at your sides.

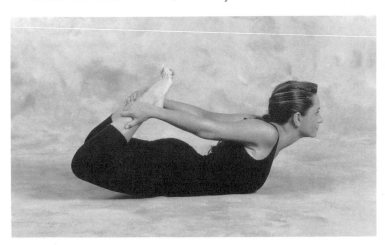

- Slowly bend your legs at the knees and bring your feet up toward your buttocks.

- Reach back with your arms and carefully take hold of first one foot and then the other. Flex your feet to make grasping them easier.

- Inhale and raise your trunk from the floor as far as possible. Lift your head and elevate your knees off the floor.

- Squeeze the buttocks. Imagine your body looking like a gently curved bow. Hold for 10 to 15 seconds.

- Slowly release the posture. Allow your chin to touch the floor and finally release your feet and return them slowly to the floor. Return to your original position. Repeat 5 times.

Stretch 5: Child's Pose

This is one of the most effective exercises for relieving menstrual cramps caused by fibroids and endometriosis. This exercise also gently stretches the lower back. It is excellent for calming anxiety and irritability. Many of my patients with menstrual cramps practice this exercise often.

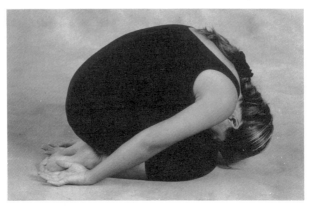

- Sit on your heels. Bring your forehead to the floor, stretching the spine as far over your head as possible.
- Close your eyes.
- Hold for as long as comfortable.

Stretch 6: Wide-Angle Pose

This is another excellent exercise for fibroid- and endometriosis-related pain and cramps. It is also useful for reducing symptoms in women with coexisting PMS and helps to relieve the congestive symptoms that occur with menstrual cramps. This stretch opens the entire pelvic region and energizes the female reproductive tract; it also relieves bloating and fluid retention in legs and feet.

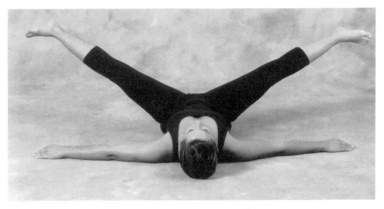

- Lie on your back with your legs against the wall and extended out in a V or an arc, and your arms extended to the sides.

- Hips should be as close to the wall as possible, buttocks on the floor. Spread legs apart as far as you can while still remaining comfortable.

- Breathing easily, hold for 1 minute, allowing the inner thighs to relax.

Suggested Reading

Bell, L., and E. Seyfer. *Gentle Yoga.* Berkeley, CA: Celestial Arts, 1987.

Couch, J., and N. Weaver. *Runner's World Yoga Book.* New York: Runner's World Books, 1979.

Folan, L. Lilias, *Yoga, and Your Life.* New York: Macmillan, 1981.

Iyengar, B. K. S. *Light on Yoga.* New York: Schocken Books, 1966.

Mittleman, R. *Yoga 28 Day Exercise Plan.* New York: Workman, 1969.

Moore, M., and M. Douglas. *Yoga.* Arcane, ME: Arcane Publications, 1967.

Singh, R. *Kundalini Yoga.* New York: White Lion Press, 1988.

Stearn, J. *Yoga, Youth and Reincarnation.* New York: Bantam, 1965.

11

Acupressure Massage

$\mathcal{A}$cupressure massage can help relieve the symptoms of bleeding, pain, and discomfort associated with fibroids and endometriosis. It is based on an ancient Oriental healing method that applies finger pressure to specific points on the skin surface to prevent and treat illness. Acupressure has had a long and distinguished history as an effective healing tool for many centuries and is often used along with herbs to promote the healing of disease.

Though Oriental medicine does not recognize the diagnoses of fibroids and endometriosis, the symptoms of these conditions can nonetheless be alleviated by relieving the imbalances that they cause in the body, specifically in the flow of life energy, or *chi*. Chi is different from, yet similar to, electromagnetic energy. According to this view, health is a state in which the chi is equally distributed throughout the body and is present in sufficient amounts. This occurs when there is a proper balance of yin (female) and yang (male) forces in the body. Chi, or life energy, is thought to energize all the cells and tissues of the body.

Oriental medicine believes that chi runs through the body in channels called *meridians*. When working in a healthy manner, these channels distribute the energy evenly throughout the body, sometimes on the surface of the skin and at times deep inside the body, in the organs. When the energy flow in a meridian is blocked or stopped, disease occurs. As a result, the internal organs that correspond to the meridians can show symptoms of disease. Stimulating the points on the skin surface can correct the meridian flow. Hand massage can treat these points easily. Pressing specific acupressure points creates changes on two levels. On the physical level, acupressure affects muscular tension, blood circulation, and other physiological functions. On a more subtle level, traditional Oriental medicine believes that acupressure, as well as acupuncture, helps to build the body's life energy to promote healing. When the normal flow of energy through the body is resumed, the body is believed to heal itself spontaneously.

Interestingly, a medical study using acupuncture for the treatment of menstrual cramps and pain was reported in the medical literature in 1987. This study was done by Dr. Joseph Helms, a family practitioner in Berkeley, California. In his study, 43 women were divided into four groups. All these women were using medication to control menstrual pain. One group of women received treatment with the acupuncture points necessary to control the menstrual pain symptoms. The other three groups received either false acupuncture treatment or no treatment. At the end of this 12-month study, 90 percent of those receiving real acupuncture treatment reported rapid and significant symptom relief. This included relief of cramping, nausea, back pain, headaches, and fluid retention. In contrast, only 36 percent of the women who received the false acupuncture treatments said that they noted symptom relief. Other physicians using acupuncture and acupressure to treat fibroids and endometriosis symptoms note similar results. Good results are more likely to occur in women with mild to moderate symptoms. Acupressure may not be as effective in women with more severe and advanced cases; these women may need to use Western medical treatments along with a variety of self-help therapies.

In any case, acupressure has much to offer the woman suffering from fibroids or endometriosis. I suggest you try the following exercises to see if you find some that work for you.

Following the simple instructions, either you or a friend can stimulate the acupressure points through finger pressure. It is safe, painless, and does not require the use of needles. You can do this without the years of specialized training needed for the proper insertion of acupuncture needles.

How to Perform Acupressure

Acupressure should be done by yourself or by a friend, when you are relaxed. The room should be warm and quiet. Hands should be clean and nails trimmed to avoid bruising. If the hands are cold, warm them in water.

Work on the side of the body that has the most discomfort. If both sides are equally uncomfortable, choose whichever one you want. Working on one side seems to relieve the symptoms on both sides; energy or information appears to transfer from one side to the other.

Hold each indicated point with a steady pressure for 1 to 3 minutes. Apply pressure slowly with the tips or balls of the fingers. Make sure your hand is comfortable. Place several fingers over the area of the point. If you feel resistance or tension in the area to which you are applying pressure, you may want to push a little harder. However, if your hand starts to feel tense or tired, lighten the pressure a bit. Breathe gently while doing each exercise.

The acupressure point may feel somewhat tender. This means the energy pathway or meridian is blocked. During the treatment, the tenderness in the point should slowly go away. You may also have a subjective feeling of energy radiating from this point into the body. Many patients describe this sensation as very pleasant. Don't worry if you don't feel it—not everyone does. The main goal is relief from your symptoms.

To find the correct acupressure point, look in the photograph accompanying the exercise. Each point corresponds to specific points on the acupressure meridians. Massage the points once a day or more during the time that you have symptoms.

Exercise 1: Balances the Entire Reproductive System

This exercise is used to balance the energy of the female reproductive tract and alleviate all menstrual complaints. It also relieves pelvic and abdominal discomfort and low back pain, which are very common complaints in women with fibroids and endometriosis.

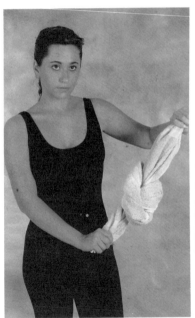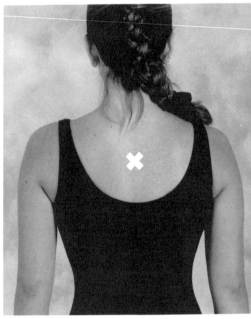

Equipment: This exercise uses a knotted hand towel to put pressure on hard-to-reach areas of the back. Place the knotted towel on these points while your two hands are on other points. This increases your ability to unblock the energy pathways of your body.

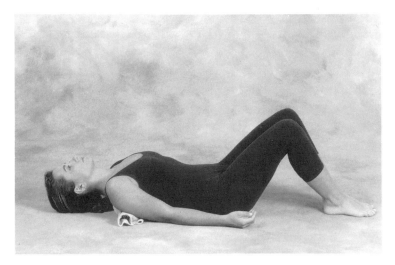

- Lie on the floor with your knees up. As you lie down, place the towel between your shoulder blades on the spine. Hold each step for 1 to 3 minutes.

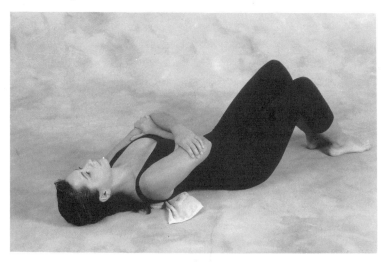

- Cross your arms over your chest. Press your thumbs against the right and left inside upper arms.

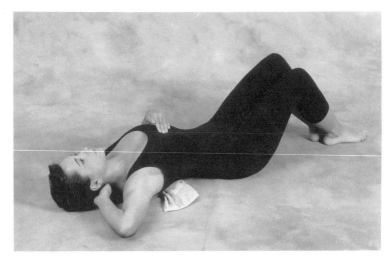

- Left hand holds point at the base of the sternum (breastbone). Right hand holds point at the base of the head (at the junction of the spine and the skull).

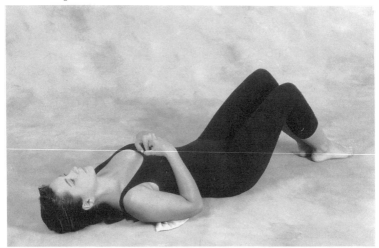

- Interlace your fingers. Place them below your breasts. Fingertips should press directly against the body.

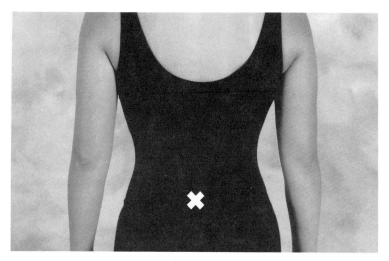

- Move the knotted towel along the spine to the waistline.

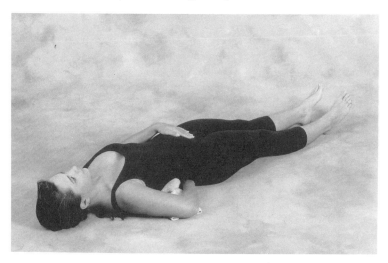

- Left hand should be placed at the top of the pubic bone, pressing down. Right hand holds point on tailbone.

Exercise 2: Relieves Cramps, Bloating, Fluid Retention, Weight Gain

This sequence balances the points on the spleen meridian, used in acupressure to relieve menstrual cramps and pelvic and abdominal discomfort associated with fibroids and endometriosis. Stimulation of these points also relieves premenstrual bloating and fluid retention and helps minimize weight gain in the period leading up to menstruation. The spleen meridian also helps regulate heavy menstrual bleeding.

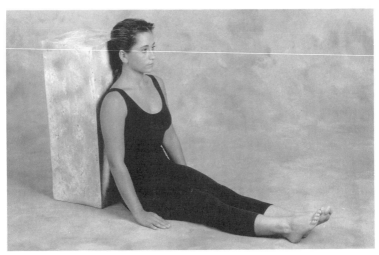

- Sit up and prop your back against a chair, or lie down and put your lower legs on a chair. Hold each step for 1 to 3 minutes.

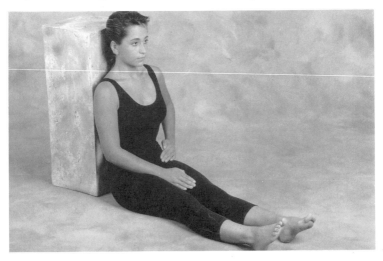

- Left hand is placed in the crease of the groin where you bend your leg, one-third to one-half way between the hip bone and the outside edge of the pubic bone. Right hand holds a spot 2 to 3 inches above the knee.

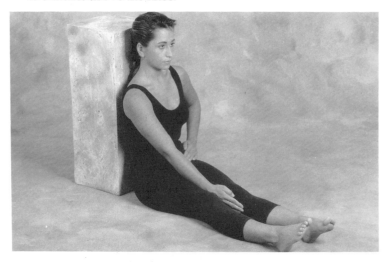

- Left hand remains in the crease of the groin. Right hand holds point below inner part of knee. To find the point, follow the curve of the bone just below the knee. Hold the underside of the curve with your fingers.

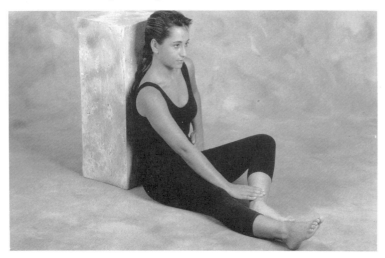

- Left hand remains in the crease of the groin. Right hand holds the inside of the shin. To find this point, go four fingerwidths above the ankle bone. The point is just above the top finger.

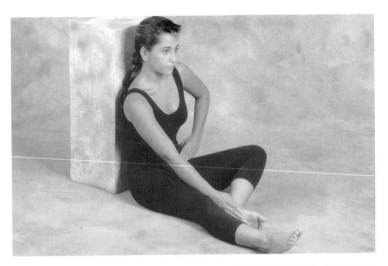

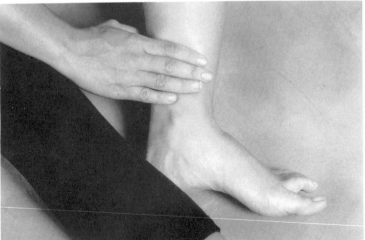

- Left hand remains in the crease of the groin. Right hand holds the edge of the instep. To find the point, follow the big toe bone up until you hit a knobby, prominent small bone.

- Left hand remains in the crease of the groin. Right hand holds the big toe over the nail, front and back of the toe.

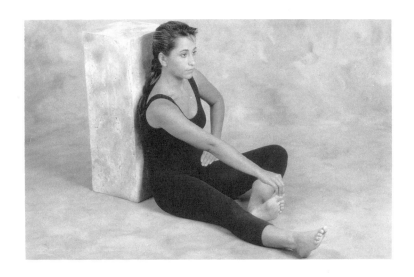

Exercise 3: Relieves Low Back Pain and Cramps

This exercise relieves menstrual cramps and low back pain by balancing points on the bladder meridian. This meridian relieves symptoms by balancing the energy of the female reproductive tract. These points are also used in Oriental medicine to relieve PMS symptoms, pelvic tension, and urinary problems, which often coexist with fibroids and endometriosis.

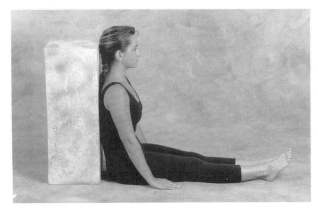

- Sit on the floor and prop your back against a wall or a heavy piece of furniture. Hold each step for 1 to 3 minutes.

- *Alternative method:* Lie on the floor and put your lower legs over the seat of a chair. Follow the exercise from that position.

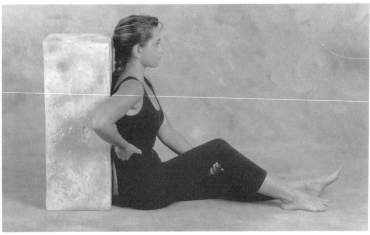

- Place left hand 1 inch above the waist on the muscle to the left side of the spine (muscle will feel firm and ropelike). Place right hand behind crease of the left knee.

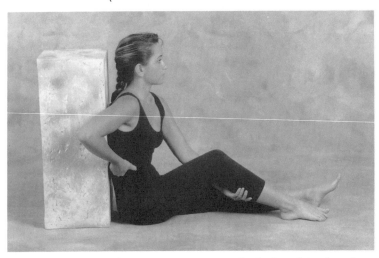

- Left hand stays in the same position. Right hand is placed on the center of the back of the left calf. This is just below the fullest part of the calf.

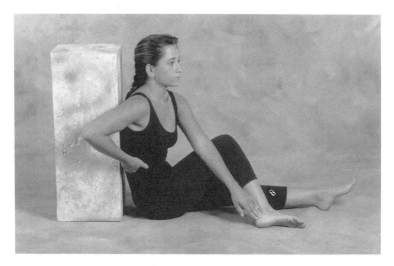

- Left hand remains 1 inch above the waist on the muscle to the side of the spine. Right hand is placed just below the ankle bone on the outside of the left heel.

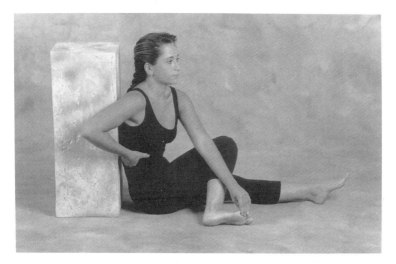

- Left hand remains 1 inch above the waist on the muscle to the side of the spine. Right hand holds the front and back of the left little toe at the nail.

Exercise 4: Relieves Nausea

This exercise relieves the nausea and digestive symptoms that often occur with cramps and low back pain. Endometriosis can also directly cause digestive symptoms when endometrial implants grow into the colon or, less frequently, into the small intestine. Fibroids can cause digestive symptoms when the tumors grow so large that they put direct pressure on the colon.

- Lie on the floor or sit up. Hold these points 1 to 3 minutes.

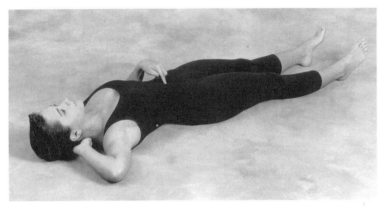

- Left index finger is placed in navel and pointed slightly toward the head. Right hand holds point at the base of the head.

Exercise 5: Relieves Menstrual Fatigue and Stress

This sequence of points relieves the fatigue that women experience just prior to the onset of the menstrual period. For many women, tiredness may last through the first few days of menstruation. Women with heavy menstrual bleeding due to fibroids and endometriosis may tire easily because of blood loss. This exercise can also relieve menstrual anxiety and depression, helpful to women suffering from significant stress in their lives. The second step in this sequence has traditionally been forbidden for use by pregnant women after their first trimester.

- Sit up and prop your back against a chair. Hold each step for 1 to 3 minutes.

- Left hand holds point at the base of the ball of the right foot. This point is located between the two pads of the foot.

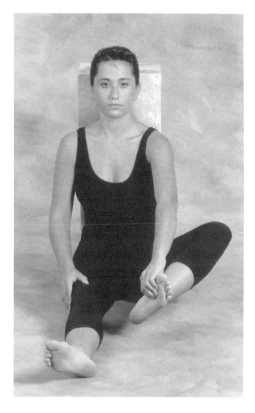

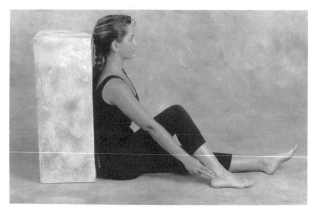

- Left hand holds the point midway between the inside of the right anklebone and the Achilles tendon. The Achilles tendon is located at the back of the ankle.

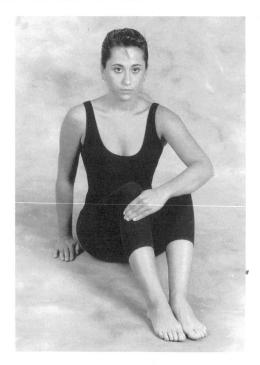

- Left hand holds point below right knee. This point is located four fingerwidths below the kneecap toward the outside of the shinbone. It is sensitive to the touch in many people.

Exercise 6: Relieves Cramps, Digestive Symptoms, and Menstrual Irregularity

This exercise stimulates conception vessel points on the front of the body. These points help relieve the pain of menstrual cramps caused by fibroids and endometriosis as well as constipation, which can accompany these problems. These points are also used to help treat menstrual irregularity.

* Sit or lie in a comfortable position.

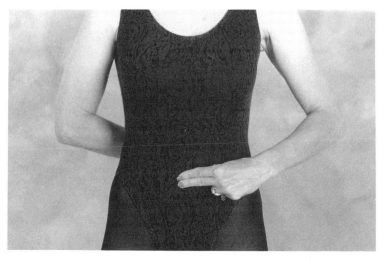

* Place your fingertips on the point two fingerwidths below the navel and hold.

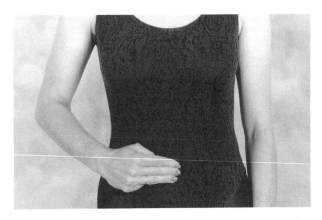

- Move your fingertips to the point four fingerwidths below the navel and hold.

Exercise 7: Relieves
Heavy Menstrual Bleeding

This sequence of points is important for the treatment of heavy menstrual flow, which can accompany fibroids and endometriosis. Heavy menstrual bleeding is also a common cause of chronic fatigue and tiredness. This exercise involves the stimulation of points on the spleen meridian, which affect blood formation and menstrual problems.

- Sit upright on a chair. Hold each step for 1 to 3 minutes.

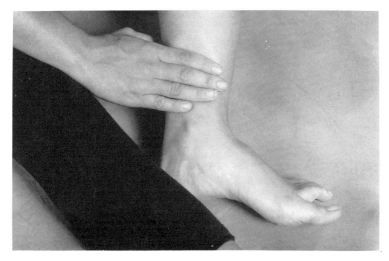

- Right hand holds point four fingerwidths above the ankle bone.

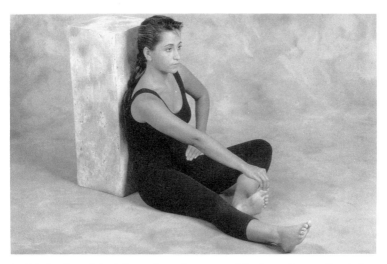

- Right hand holds point above and below the nail of the big toe.

Suggested Reading

The Academy of Traditional Chinese Medicine. *An Outline of Chinese Acupuncture.* New York: Pergamon Press, 1975.

Bauer, C. *Acupressure for Women.* Freedom, CA: The Crossing Press, 1987.

Chang, S. *The Complete Book of Acupuncture.* Berkeley, CA: Celestial Arts, 1976.

Gach, M. R., and C. Marco. *Acu-Yoga.* Tokyo: Japan Publications, 1981.

Houston, F. M. *The Healing Benefits of Acupressure.* New Canaan, CT: Keats Publishing, 1974.

Kenyon, J. *Acupressure Techniques.* Rochester, VT: Healing Arts Press, 1980.

Nickel, D. J. *Acupressure for Athletes.* New York: Henry Holt, 1984.

Pendleton, B., and B. Mehling. *Relax With Self-Therap/Ease.* Englewood Cliffs, NJ: Prentice-Hall, 1984.

Teeguarden, I. *Acupressure Way of Health: Jin Shin Do.* Tokyo: Japan Publications, 1978.

12

Treating Fibroids & Endometriosis with Drugs

$\mathcal{F}$ibroids and endometriosis may have similar symptoms, but medical treatments of them differ. Drugs and hormonal therapies have been the mainstay of the Western medical response to endometriosis for the past 30 to 40 years. For the treatment of fibroids, fewer drugs are effective, and surgery has traditionally been a more effective option. However, in recent years, several drugs have been used effectively to treat fibroids.

A few of these medications are available to women over the counter, while other, stronger drugs need a doctor's prescription and require careful monitoring. Some medications—such as narcotics, birth control pills, male hormones and progestins, diuretics, and muscle relaxants—have been around for a long time and have been the traditional drug treatments for endometriosis. Others, specifically the prescription antiprostaglandins, synthetic male hormones, and GnRH (gonadotropin-releasing hormone) analogs, have only been available for use in treating endometriosis (or fibroids, if GnRH analogs are used) for the past 15 years. These new drug therapies have provided women with a major source of symptom relief and are commonly used today.

Over-the-Counter Medications

Many women with endometriosis use over-the-counter pain and cramp medications because they mistakenly believe they are treating simple menstrual cramps. These products may provide some relief in the earliest stages of endometriosis, if symptoms are mild. As endometriosis progresses in severity, symptom relief from these drugs may not continue. One of the oldest cramp-relief medications is simply aspirin. Interestingly, aspirin is a mild prostaglandin inhibitor, although it is only one-thirtieth as strong as the new antiprostaglandin drugs. The F_2 Alpha prostaglandins cause uterine contractions when present in the reproductive tract in high concentrations around the time of menstruation. In addition to worsening pain and cramps, these prostaglandins may accelerate the spread of endometriosis by causing retrograde menstruation. Always take aspirin with food to avoid stomach discomfort and use it with great caution if you have a preexisting peptic ulcer or a tendency toward heartburn, because it can worsen or reactivate symptoms.

Another more recently available prostaglandin inhibitor is ibuprofen. This drug is sold over the counter as Advil or Nuprin, in 200-milligram tablets. The dose commonly used for menstrual pain and cramps is two tablets, or 400 milligrams, taken every six hours. Like aspirin, ibuprofen should be taken with food as it can cause gastrointestinal upset.

Some over-the-counter remedies for menstrual pain contain several drugs in combination. Products such as Midol, Pamprin, and a number of others contain aspirin, an antispasmodic to relieve muscle tension, caffeine (which causes widening in the diameter of peripheral blood vessels), and sometimes a diuretic for relief of congestive symptoms. Like the mild antiprostaglandins, they may be used frequently with early-stage, undiagnosed endometriosis. Be careful to follow the dosage instructions on the bottle; if used in excess, many of these drugs can cause undesired side effects. Aspirin can cause gastric distress; caffeine can make people nervous and jittery and may also upset the stomach by increasing gastric acid secretion. Pamabrom, a diuretic agent used in several products, can lead to loss of minerals, like all diuretics. Another commonly used ingredient in these products is pyrilamine, an antihistamine. Antihistamines are normally used to relieve symptoms of allergylike nasal congestion. They also have the tendency to cause drowsiness or sedation and are used in menstrual remedies for these sedative effects. Although the doses used are small, some women who are sensitive may encounter side effects.

Prescription Medications

A number of medications for the treatment of fibroids and endometriosis can only be prescribed by a physician. These are generally used to control moderate to severe symptoms.

Prostaglandin Inhibitors. These drugs, also called nonsteroidal anti-inflammatory agents, are a relatively new class of prescription drugs for the treatment of menstrual cramps, as well as the pain and cramps caused by endometriosis. They tend to be effective in relieving the symptoms of primary spasmodic dysmenorrhea and may help limit the spread of endometriosis through retrograde menstruation, especially when triggered with severe uterine contractions. For many women, the use of these drugs can make the difference between being able to function during the menstrual period and being so incapacitated by pain that they must spend one or two days in bed.

These medications are particularly useful for endometriosis and cramps, since they have both anti-inflammatory and pain-killing properties. These drugs were originally developed for the treatment of arthritis and are primarily available by prescription; they include Motrin, Naprosyn, Anaprox, and Ponstel. Ibuprofen (Advil, Nuprin) is available by prescription in higher dosage levels as Motrin. These drugs must be used carefully, however, since they can cause gastrointestinal bleeding and peptic ulcer disease or even reactivate a preexisting ulcer. Approximately 10 percent of women who use these medications report digestive symptoms, including heartburn, nausea, vomiting, diarrhea, constipation, and poor digestion. To lessen the likelihood of these side effects, always take these medications with food. Report any significant digestive symptoms to your physician. Some women report other unpleasant symptoms when using prostaglandin inhibitors—drowsiness, headaches, vertigo, dizziness, rashes, blurred vision, anemia, edema, and heart palpitations. Avoid using these drugs with aspirin, since both can cause gastrointestinal bleeding and irritation.

Narcotics. Narcotics such as codeine are very effective painkillers and can certainly numb the discomfort of endometriosis or menstrual cramps. They do, however, have significant side effects and don't reverse the underlying cause of the menstrual cramps or halt the spread of endometrial implants. The side effects of narcotics commonly include constipation, nausea, and drowsiness. Be sure to avoid driving your car when using a narcotic painkiller because you may fall asleep at the wheel. Other painkillers like Darvon or relaxants like Valium are also prescribed. Though Valium is an effective relaxant, it can also cause drowsiness and sedation. All of these drugs can be addictive. Women who use them on an ongoing basis often find that they need higher doses and more frequent usage in order to continue a beneficial therapeutic effect. I generally recommend that women use these drugs very infrequently and only if symptoms are particularly severe.

Birth Control Pills. These drugs have been the primary treatment for endometriosis since the 1950s. Many physicians still prescribe birth control pills as the treatment of choice for endometriosis. Birth control pills contain estrogen and a synthetic progesterone (or progestin) in varying doses. The estrogen and progestin in the birth control pills shut down your body's natural production of hormones. The hormones in the medication trick your pituitary and hypothalamus into thinking your ovaries have produced high levels of hormones. As a result, the hypothalamus and pituitary stop secreting the hormones—FSH (follicle-stimulating hormone) and LH (luteinizing hormone)—that trigger ovarian function.

The pill also creates a state of pseudopregnancy, because it contains the same hormones found in high levels in women who are pregnant. The pills are given over a 12-month period to simulate the 9 months that women are pregnant and 3 months spent breast feeding, which also suppresses normal menstrual cycles. This year-long vacation from regular menstrual cycles can reduce endometriosis symptoms. Because the birth control pills prevent ovulation, they decrease the prostaglandin accumulation during the second half of the menstrual cycle. Prostaglandin accumulation has been linked to menstrual pain and cramps. The levels of estrogen and progestin in the birth control pills also cause lighter menstrual flow, a benefit for women with endometriosis who tend to have heavy bleeding and spotting.

The use of a low-estrogen-dose birth control pill is very important in order to reduce menstruation. The hormones used in the pill alter the endometrium (lining of the uterus) to create abnormal cells that do not cause pelvic implants, even if there is retrograde menstruation. Low-dose birth control pills currently contain less than 35 micrograms of estrogen. They are definitely preferred over high-dose estrogen pills, which can stimulate the growth of endometrial implants. As explained earlier, estrogen can trigger the acceleration and spread of endometrial growths. Thus, dosage is very important. It is important to understand that although low-dose pills can reduce pain and other symptoms of endometriosis, they do not eliminate the implants themselves.

Low-dose birth control pills are best used by young women in their teens and twenties who suffer from severe menstrual cramps and are at high risk of developing endometriosis. Other candidates for the birth control pill include women with diagnosed endometriosis who have just given birth and have not been on other previous therapy for endometriosis, such as the drug Danazol (discussed later in this chapter). For these women, the oral contraceptive may help prevent the recurrence of endometriosis symptoms as well as prevent another pregnancy, if that is desired. Birth control pills can also be used by women who have had previous drug or surgical treatment for endometriosis, and don't wish to become pregnant. In all these cases, the birth control pill is used in the standard way: Women are given three weeks of hormones, taking one pill per day, followed by a week of rest with no hormonal intake.

Many women, however, should not take birth control pills as a treatment for endometriosis. These include women with coexisting fibroid tumors, a history of blood clots, high blood pressure, liver or gall bladder disease, preexisting breast or uterine cancer, or those who smoke. Some women with milder cases of endometriosis find that their symptoms diminish with the use of the pill, but they experience uncomfortable side effects such as weight gain, fluid retention, breast tenderness, PMS mood changes, and headaches. In some cases, the side effects are so uncomfortable that the birth control pills must be discontinued.

Depo-Provera. This is a synthetic progesterone used like the birth control pill to cause pseudopregnancy. Like the pill, it creates a vacation from the monthly surge of natural hormones that trigger and accelerate the spread of endometriosis. Women on Depo-Provera experience a prolonged time without menstrual periods or only light bleeding and spotting. During Depo-Provera treatment, endometriosis symptoms diminish, but aberrant endometrial tissue will not shrink and melt away. Thus, once the treatment ends, the implants can continue to grow and spread.

Unlike the birth control pill, which is taken orally on a daily basis, Depo-Provera is injected into the muscle and acts on a long-term basis. The first injection is followed by another treatment four to eight weeks later. Subsequent treatments are given every six to ten weeks, for one year, mimicking a normal pregnancy and breast-feeding period. Possible side effects include bloating, fluid retention, headaches, pelvic pain, and fatigue. In research studies done on dogs, Depo-Provera was also found to cause breast tumors. Depo-Provera is probably not a good choice for women who want to become pregnant shortly after completing their course of treatment. The body can take a year or more to eliminate all traces of this drug, once active treatment has ceased. As a result, ovulation may be suppressed and fertility hampered for a year following treatment. Depo-Provera may, however, be a good drug for women who cannot tolerate the more commonly used drugs for endometriosis, like Danazol, because of their side effects.

Danazol. This is one of the most popular current hormonal therapies for endometriosis. It has also been used to treat fibrocystic breast disease, but has not been particularly useful for fibroids. Danazol, marketed as Danocrine in the United States, is a synthetic hormone derived from the male hormone testosterone. It induces a pseudomenopause by directly depressing the output of FSH (follicle-stimulating hormone) and LH (luteinizing hormone) from the pituitary and hypothalamus and lowering estrogen production by the ovaries. Because of this effect on the endocrine glands, Danazol is called a gonadotropin inhibitor. It also acts to alter the metabolism of estrogen and progesterone and to block the estrogen and progesterone receptors in the endometrial implants. These changes lead to both relief of endometriosis symptoms and shrinkage of the implants. Large masses and adhesions or scar tissue actually disappear. This offers tremendous benefit to women with endometriosis, 85 percent of whom report significant relief. Danazol may cause the regression of fibrocystic breast lesions and can be beneficial in treating this disease.

Treatment is generally instituted for 6 to 12 months, depending on the severity of the disease. Danazol is generally prescribed in doses between 400 and 800 milligrams, often in two daily doses, one to be taken at night and one during the day. The drug generally reduces estrogen to levels low enough to stop menstruation. Often this reduction takes several months, and many women notice light menstrual bleeding for the first few months.

Danazol does have drawbacks, however. For one thing, it does not cure endometriosis. One survey of 180 women conducted by the Endometriosis Association in Milwaukee, Wisconsin, reported that more than 50 percent of women surveyed who had taken Danazol either had no symptom relief or had a recurrence of symptoms immediately after stopping the drug. In another report in medical literature, 20 percent taking the drug noted a recurrence of endometrial symptoms within a year after stopping Danazol therapy. This incidence continues to increase with time.

Another problem that many women using Danazol encounter is unpleasant side effects. While Danazol itself does not cause masculinization, it decreases estrogen levels enough that a woman's natural male hormonal response is accentuated. This can lead to acne, abnormal hair growth, increased oiliness of the skin or hair, weight gain, decrease in breast size, deepening of the voice, and even rarely, clitoral hypertrophy. These masculinizing effects are, unfortunately, not always reversible. Due to the decline in the estrogen levels, women on Danazol may also have menopause symptoms such as hot flashes, night sweats, and vaginal dryness. Other unpleasant side effects include bloating, fluid retention, weight gain, changes in liver function, muscle cramps, headaches, dizziness, depression, and anxiety. Obviously Danazol, for all its benefits, must be carefully monitored by a physician during the course of therapy.

GnRH Analogs. These drugs, such as Lupron and Nafarelin, have been tested experimentally in recent years as another treatment for both fibroids and endometriosis. They are chemically similar to the gonadotropin-releasing hormone (GnRH or LH-RH) that triggers secretion of LH and FSH by the pituitary. The pituitary in turn regulates the ovarian output of estrogen and progesterone. The analog drugs are given by nasal spray or injection and, like Danazol, inhibit the hypothalamus-pituitary-ovarian feedback loop. As a result, FSH and LH secretion is inhibited and estrogen levels decrease. Also like Danazol, these drugs produce relief of endometriosis and shrink endometrial implants and fibroids. GnRH analogs have also been used for the treatment of other diseases for which suppression of estrogen is important, such as ovarian cysts.

One benefit of the GnRH analogs is that they don't have masculinizing side effects like Danazol. They do, however, produce the typical symptoms of menopause—hot flashes, mood swings, back and muscle pain, and headaches. They also increase the long-term risk of osteoporosis by lowering the estrogen level and increasing calcium excretion from the body. The side effects can be quite unpleasant; I have had a number of younger women see me in consultation purely to work with the menopausal side effects that the analogs cause.

In summary, many drug therapies are available for treatment of endometriosis, and several may also help treat fibroids. Though many of these offer only symptomatic relief, certain drugs can shrink fibroid tumors and endometrial implants. Still, none of these therapies is curative and, in many cases, they cause unpleasant side effects. The stronger drugs must be prescribed and carefully monitored by a physician. I always recommend that women on drug therapy for fibroids or endometriosis also follow a complete self-help program to regulate and balance their hormonal levels, to build up their immune system to limit the spread of the tissue damage, and to control emotional stress. These self-help therapies, in combination with judicious use of medication, can provide effective relief for many women suffering from endometriosis and, with the use of GnRH, fibroids.

Women with endometriosis should not use birth control pills if they have any of the following symptoms:

Fibroid tumors

Blood clots in the legs, pelvis, or lungs

High blood pressure

Liver or gall bladder disease

History of breast or uterine cancer

Use of cigarettes or tobacco products

Common Side Effects of the Birth Control Pill
Weight gain, fluid retention, bloating
Breast tenderness
Premenstrual syndrome
Mood changes
Headaches

Side Effects of Danazol
Acne, oily hair and skin
Abnormal hair growth
Weight gain
Decrease in breast size
Deepening of the voice
Clitoral hypertrophy
Hot flashes, night sweats
Vaginal atrophy
Vaginitis
Fluid retention, bloating
Changes in liver function
Muscle cramps
Headaches, dizziness

Medications for Endometriosis

Over-the-Counter Medications
Aspirin
Ibuprofen (Advil, Nuprin)
Pamprin

Prescription Drugs
Antiprostaglandin Inhibitors
Motrin
Anaprox
Midol
Ponstel
Naprosyn

Narcotics
Codeine
Darvon

Hormonal Therapies
Birth control pills
Depo-Provera
Danazol
Lupron
Nafarelin

Medications for Fibroids

Prescription Drugs
Hormonal Therapies
Lupron
Nafarelin

Side Effects of GnRH Analogs
Hot flashes, night sweats
Vaginal atrophy
Mood swings
Increased calcium excretion
Osteoporosis
Breast tenderness
High blood pressure
Digestive changes
Anemia
Headaches, dizziness
Increase in urinary frequency

Surgery for Relief of Fibroids & Endometriosis

13

*M*any women with fibroids and endometriosis never need surgery, primarily because these conditions are not causing severe physical symptoms. Many women with mild to moderate symptoms may handle the disease process quite effectively through a self-help program or drug and hormonal therapies. Remember that both problems may become less severe with the onset of menopause when the hormonal levels decrease. Both fibroids and endometriosis are stimulated by high levels of estrogen. Conservative management may allow a woman to preserve her uterus and avoid the physical and emotional stress of surgery.

However, for some women with fibroids or endometriosis, surgery is unavoidable and necessary. In this chapter I discuss the surgical techniques commonly used to treat these conditions, as well as their indications and risks.

Surgery for Fibroid Tumors

Current Western medicine offers two surgical options for treatment of fibroids. A myomectomy allows the preservation of the uterus, while a hysterectomy necessitates the removal of the uterus along with the fibroid tumors.

Myomectomy. This procedure removes the fibroid tumors while preserving the uterus. Younger and mid-life women find this an attractive surgical option because it preserves their childbearing abilities and often increases sexual pleasure and intensity. Of the younger women whose infertility is caused by fibroids (as many as 10 percent of all cases of infertility), up to 54 percent conceive following a myomectomy. Also, the rate of spontaneous abortion due to fibroids drops substantially following myomectomy.

The surgeon may perform a myomectomy through a vaginal incision or an abdominal incision, depending on the location of the fibroids. Many surgeons will not perform a myomectomy when the uterine size is too big or the woman has too many fibroids. Though the number and size of the fibroids are not an absolute technical deterrent in themselves, removal of a large number of these benign tumors may be beyond the scope of many surgeons. The number of fibroids found once the uterus is exposed in surgery can be astonishing. Several dozen fibroids are not unusual, and numbers as high as 200 have been reported by surgeons. These can range from tiny seedling tumors to large tumors weighing many pounds. If you want to consider a myomectomy, find a surgeon who is comfortable and very experienced with this technique.

Having an experienced surgeon also helps minimize side effects from the procedure. Complications can include blood loss from the surgery and postoperative scarring or adhesions. Postoperative adhesions can themselves impair fertility.

Some surgeons work to control adhesions with microsurgical techniques, using instruments that cause minimal tissue damage and controlling the amount of bleeding carefully so that very little blood remains at the surgery site. This helps minimize the development of postoperative inflammation and adhesions. The use of the laser instead of traditional surgical tools has been pioneered in recent years. Using a laser does not change the basic surgical procedure, since the surgeon must still open up the patient and cut out the fibroids. However, surgeons skilled in the use of the laser can do the procedure with less blood loss during surgery. The amount of postoperative pain may be lessened, too. This is obviously of great benefit to the patient, as it may permit more comfortable healing.

Myomectomy may not be a definitive cure of fibroids for many women. Based on follow-up medical studies, women face a 15 to 45 percent risk of growth of new fibroids, which may necessitate further surgery. The mortality rate for both myomectomies and hysterectomies, however, is nearly identical—on the order of 1 to 2 percent. For a woman who wishes to preserve her uterus, myomectomy offers a viable option if surgery must be performed.

Hysterectomy. This procedure is the definitive cure for fibroids, because the entire uterus, along with the fibroids, is removed during the operation. Obviously, with a hysterectomy the recurrence of fibroids is not an issue.

Fibroids is one of the most common reasons for this procedure to be done in the United States; approximately one-third of all hysterectomies are done for fibroid treatment. In my opinion, some of these hysterectomies probably don't need to be done. Some doctors suggest a hysterectomy if the uterus is greater than a 12- to 16-week-size pregnant uterus, even in women with mild or no symptoms. In the absence of symptoms, size of the uterus alone is not a good reason for this operation. If the fibroid is not pressing on the bladder, rectum, or another pelvic structure, a woman may go for years without having any symptoms at all. Eventually these tumors will likely shrink and may even disappear with menopause.

Some women with very large asymptomatic fibroids may wish to have a hysterectomy for cosmetic reasons, if the fibroids are causing noticeable protrusion or bulging of the abdominal wall. If your physician suggests a hysterectomy for fibroids that are symptom-free, I suggest that you get a second opinion from another physician in your area known to be more conservative in his or her management.

Strong indications for a hysterectomy include the following:

- Extremely heavy bleeding that causes anemia or significant lifestyle problems.

- Severe pelvic pain and menstrual cramps.

- Rapidly enlarging uterine size with worsening pelvic pressure. In a postmenopausal woman, this requires careful evaluation because, on rare occasions, it may indicate a malignancy in the uterus. (However, less than one-third of 1 percent of all fibroids are found to have malignant properties.)

- Pressure symptoms causing changes in normal bladder and bowel functions, such as increased urinary frequency or constipation.

If you have any of these symptoms, a hysterectomy may be the correct and even necessary therapy to treat your fibroids. For women who do not wish to preserve their fertility and childbearing capability, the decision to have a hysterectomy for one of these reasons may be a noncontroversial choice.

Before agreeing to have a hysterectomy, be informed about all the risks and benefits of the procedure. It is important that women take responsibility for their bodies and learn as much as they can about the surgery. Talk to your doctor. Good communication is a crucial part of a good doctor-patient relationship. Remember, this is one of the most important relationships that you will ever have in your life. Your physician plays a major role in helping to preserve your health and well-being. In the case of a hysterectomy, your physician will be opening up your body surgically. Be sure you feel comfortable with your doctor. Ask about the emotional and physical risks to you, how long recovery will take, and how you can expect to feel afterward. Remember, your physician has an enormous backlog of knowledge, because he or she has probably seen the effects of the surgery on thousands of other patients.

As with a myomectomy, complications may include blood

loss. In fact, if blood loss is substantial, a blood transfusion during surgery may be necessary. Infections at the site of the surgical incisions, or at other sites like the bladder or lung, may occur also postoperatively. Often, women are simply not prepared for how they will feel after surgery. In my practice, I have had many patients come for consultation after a hysterectomy. While many women recover quickly, some do not. I have had patients who were shocked at how tired and depressed they felt for months after surgery. Though their surgeons had warned them that they should not lift heavy items and should avoid rigorous physical activity during the postoperative period, they received no warning that their quality of life might suffer, that they might feel more emotional and upset, or that their sexual enjoyment might diminish after removal of their uterus. Often the women who seek me out after a hysterectomy are looking to regain their presurgical zest and well-being. They are looking for therapies based on lifestyle changes, such as an optimal nutritional program and stress management, to experience once again a sense of good health and well-being. The self-help chapters of this book describe many of the techniques I have found to be helpful for such patients.

Surgery for Endometriosis

With endometriosis, the goals of surgery are to relieve pain or to restore fertility and, ideally, prevent recurrence of the disease. Depending on the severity of the disease and the age of the patient, the physician may recommend either conservative surgery or more extensive surgery. Conservative surgery allows the preservation of the patient's reproductive organs while removing the endometriosis implants; more extensive surgery removes both the endometriosis implants and the reproductive organs.

Conservative Surgery. This involves the removal of the implants at the time the actual diagnosis is made by a laparoscopy. As discussed in Chapter 2, the laparoscope is an instrument that allows visualization of the pelvic cavity and the reproductive organs. Once the implants, adhesions, endometrial cysts, or other changes typical of endometriosis are visualized, treatment can be initiated at once. In many cases, this prevents the need for a second, follow-up surgical procedure after diagnosis. Treatment consists of destroying the implants by the use of a laser or electrocautery. Either technique can remove scarring or adhesions, implants, and small ovarian cysts.

Some physicians prefer laser therapy because it involves less blood loss, less thermal damage to the tissues by the instrument, and fewer postoperative adhesions. Also, cautery should be avoided in treating the fallopian tubes or bladder because of the risk of burning these tissues. However, in the hands of an experienced surgeon, cautery is also a very effective and useful technique. When faced with a choice, women should seek out physicians who are skilled at laparoscopic surgery. The doctor's technical proficiency in performing either technique is paramount in determining how good the results will be. To improve the cure rate, many physicians combine surgery with drug therapy like Danazol. Drug therapy is often given either pre- or postoperatively for a period of time to further reduce the risk of recurrence.

There are women for whom laparoscopic surgery is not a good option. Women with extensive endometriosis, many adhesions, involvement of the bowel or urinary tract, large endometrial cysts, or extensive disease in the ovaries may need more radical surgery. These problems are often beyond the scope of laser or cautery treatment and may require a larger incision and removal of the reproductive organs, as well as destruction of the implant and scar tissue.

How successful is conservative surgery? In those women who undergo surgery primarily to restore fertility, the success of the treatment depends on the extent of the disease process. Medical studies have shown that women with moderate endometriosis have a 50 to 60 percent pregnancy rate after surgery, while women with severe endometriosis have a 30 to 40 percent chance of conceiving. The recurrence rate after surgery is fairly high. One percent of patients have a recurrence of active endometriosis within the first year following surgery, while the three- and five-year recurrence rates are 13 and 40 percent, respectively. Some women will eventually require a second laparoscopic procedure or even a total abdominal hysterectomy as treatment for recurrence.

Extensive Surgery. Surgeons often recommend more extensive surgery to women in their thirties and forties who have more severe disease and to women for whom fertility is not an issue. A woman in her middle to late thirties and forties who has completed or does not desire childbearing may elect to undergo major surgery, in which the surgeon opens the abdomen and removes the uterus along with all visible implants and adhesions.

To avoid an early menopause, the surgeon should try to spare the ovaries (or at least part of one ovary, if the endometriosis has attached itself to these glands) if at all possible. A premature surgical menopause can be difficult for women to tolerate when the ovaries are entirely removed. Symptoms such as hot flashes and vaginal dryness can be quite severe. Also, the risk of developing osteoporosis over time is greater in these women. Further, there is a slight chance of reactivating the endometriosis in women who had a total hysterectomy once they begin hormonal replacement therapy, because estrogen stimulates the growth of the implants. It may be impossible to remove all the microscopic implants during the operation, thus leaving behind tissue that can reactivate under hormonal stimulation. This can be a double-edged sword for younger women who don't want to suffer from hot flashes, yet are concerned about possible hormonal side effects.

Therefore, I strongly believe in preserving ovarian function if at all possible in women who must undergo surgery for endometriosis. Unfortunately, complete removal of the ovaries, tubes, and uterus is common, particularly if a woman is in her forties. This happens even when the disease is entirely treatable by removal of only the implants and scar tissue. I recommend that women choose their surgeon carefully, with the goal of preserving as many of their reproductive organs as possible without sacrificing the best therapeutic response. If major surgery is required, it is important to speak with several doctors to learn what options are available.

14

Putting Your Program Together

*T*his book has given you a complete self-help program to help prevent and relieve your symptoms. Try the treatment options that feel most comfortable to you. You may find that certain exercise routines or stress reduction techniques feel better to you than others. If that is the case, practice the ones that bring the greatest sense of relief for your particular symptoms.

Don't get bogged down in details. Always keep in mind that your ultimate goal is relief of your fibroid or endometriosis symptoms and a general improvement in your overall health and well-being. I usually recommend beginning any self-help program slowly while you get used to the changes in lifestyle. People differ in their ability to adjust to major lifestyle changes. Though some of my patients like to eliminate their old, unhealthy habits as quickly as possible, many other women find such rapid changes in long-term habits too stressful. Find the pace that works for you.

Enjoy the program. I always tell my patients to regard their self-help program as an enjoyable adventure. The exercises and stress-reduction techniques should give you a sense of energy and well-being. The menus and food selections I've recommended in this book provide you with an opportunity to try delicious and healthful new foods.

As you do the program, don't set up unrealistic or overly strict expectations for yourself. You don't have to be perfect to get great results. Just follow the guidelines of the program as best you can and as your schedule permits.

It is not a disaster if you forget to take your vitamins occasionally or don't have time to exercise on a particular day. Don't be discouraged if you can't follow the dietary recommendations on vacations, holidays, and birthdays. Periodically review the guidelines outlined in this book and continue to adapt your lifestyle to the healthful suggestions that I've shared with you from my years of medical practice. Over time you will notice many beneficial changes.

Be your own feedback system. Your body will tell you if you are on the right track and if what you are doing is making you feel better. It will also tell you if your current diet and emotional stresses are worsening your symptoms. Remember that even moderate changes in your habits can make significant differences.

The Fibroid and Endometriosis Workbook

Fill out the workbook section of this book. The workbook questionnaires will help you determine which areas in your life have contributed the most to your symptoms and need the most improvement. Review the workbook every month or two as you follow the self-help program. The workbook will help you see the areas in which you are making the most progress, with both symptom relief and the adoption of healthier lifestyle habits. The workbook can help give you feedback in an organized and easy-to-use manner.

Diet and Nutritional Supplements

I recommend that you make all nutritional changes gradually. Many women find breakfast the easiest meal to change because it is simple and often eaten at home. To change your other meals and snacks, periodically review the list of foods to eliminate and foods to emphasize. Each month, pick a few foods that you are willing to eliminate from your diet. Try in their place the foods that help prevent and relieve fibroid and endometriosis symptoms. The recipes and menus in Chapter 5 should be very helpful; use the meal plans as helpful guidelines while you restructure your diet to suit your needs.

Vitamins, minerals, essential fatty acids, and herbal supplements can help complete your nutritional needs and speed up the healing process. Most women consider supplements an essential part of their program.

Stress-Reduction and Breathing Exercises

The stress-reduction and breathing exercises play an important role in facilitating the physical healing process. I find that all my patients heal more rapidly from almost any problem when they are calm, happy, and relaxed. The visualization exercises can help you set a blueprint in your mind for optimal health; this enables your body and mind to work together in harmony.

Begin the program by putting aside 15 to 30 minutes each day, depending on the flexibility of your schedule. Try all the stress-reduction and breathing exercises listed in this book. Choose the combination that works best for you. Practice stress management on a regular basis and be aware of your habitual breathing patterns. Both techniques will help normalize your hormonal balance, relax your uterine, pelvic, and back muscles, and release tension, giving you a more comfortable menstrual period.

You do not need to spend enormous amounts of time on these exercises. Many women are too busy, for example, to spend an hour a day meditating. Even 10 minutes out of your daily schedule can be helpful. You may find that the quietest times for you are early in the morning before you get out of bed, or late at night before going to sleep. Some women simply choose to take a break during the day. You can close the door to your office or go into your bedroom at home for 10 minutes to relax. Use the time to breathe deeply, do the visualizations, or meditate. You will be much calmer and more relaxed afterward.

Physical Exercise, Yoga, and Acupressure

You should do moderate exercise on a regular basis, at least three times a week. Aerobic exercise can improve both circulation and oxygenation to tight, constricted muscles, thereby helping you relax. It is important, however, to do your exercise routine slowly and comfortably. Frenetic exercise that is too fast-paced can push your muscles to the point of exhaustion and tense them further. Women with fibroid- or endometriosis-related pain and cramps need to keep their muscles and joints flexible and supple. To this end, try the fitness and flexibility exercises in this book.

To do the yoga stretches and acupressure massage, set aside a half-hour each day for the first week or two of your self-help program. Try all the exercises. After an initial period of exploration, choose the ones that you enjoy the most and that seem to give you the most relief. Practice them on a regular basis so that they can help to prevent and reduce your symptoms.

Conclusion

I wish to reaffirm that each of us can do a tremendous amount for ourselves to assure optimal health and well-being. By having access to information, education, and health resources, every woman can play a major role in creating her own state of good health. Practice the beneficial self-help techniques that I've outlined in this book. Follow good nutritional habits, exercise, and practice stress-reduction techniques regularly.

By combining good principles of self-care along with your regular medical care, you can enjoy the same wonderful results that my patients and I have had for a life of good health and well-being.

Health & Lifestyle Resources for Women

Magazines

The following magazines feature articles on a wide array of health and wellness topics. Strong emphasis is placed on nutrition, holistic health, natural cures and remedies, and preventive medicine. The authors of the articles include physicians, health care and nutrition professionals, and experienced freelance writers who specialize in health-related subjects.

American Health
28 West 23rd Street
New York, NY 10010
10 times/year $18.97/year

Body, Mind & Spirit
255 Hope Street
Providence, RI 02906
6 times/year $21.00/year

Let's Live
320 North Larchmont Boulevard
P.O. Box 7498
Los Angeles, CA 90004
Monthly $19.95/year

Longevity
Longevity International, Ltd
1965 Broadway
New York, NY 10023
Monthly $24.00/year

Natural Health
P.O. Box 1200
Brookline Village, MA 02147
6 times/year $24.00/year

New Age Journal
342 Wesyern Ave.
Brighton, MA 02135
7 times/year $24.00/year

Prevention
33 East Minor Street
Emmaus, PA 18098
Monthly $19.97/year

Your Health
Globe International
5401 N.W. Broken Sound Blvd.
Boca Raton, FL 33487
24 times/year $24.00/year

The following periodicals are oriented toward health and wellness but focus their articles on one specific area:

Vegetarian Journal
The Vegetarian Resource Group
P.O Box 1463
Baltimore, MD 21203
6 times/year $20.00/year

Vegetarian Times
P.O. Box 570
Oak Park, IL 60303
Monthly $23.95/year

Yoga Journal
2054 University Avenue
Berkeley, CA 94704
Monthly $21.00/year

Newsletters and Journals

The following newsletters provide excellent coverage of women's health topics:

A Friend Indeed
P.O. Box 1710
Champlain, NY 12919-1710
10 times/year $30.00/year

This newsletter is of particular interest to women in menopause or midlife, and includes a lengthy selection of letters from readers, often accompanied by responses from the editor.

Alternatives for the Health Conscious Individual
Mountain Home Publishing
2700 Cummings Lane
Kerrville, TX 78028
Monthly $39.00/year

Publishes a compilation of existing data and research on health subjects. Implies no author's or publisher's endorsement. Edited by Dr. David G. Williams.

Endometriosis Association
8585 North 76th Place
Milwaukee, WI 53203
Membership $32.00/year

A self-help organization of women with endometriosis and others interested in exchanging information about endometriosis, offering mutual support to those affected by endometriosis, educating the public and medical community about the disease, and promoting research related to endometriosis. Materials available include a newsletter for members, books, audio tapes and video tapes.

Dr. Alexander Grant's Health Gazette

P.O. Box 1786
Indianapolis, IN 46206
10 times/year $24.95/year

Provides brief summaries of articles that have appeared recently in professional journals such as *JAMA* and other newsletters such as *Nutrition Action Newsletter*. The source for each summary is identified.

Dr. Julian Whitaker's Health & Healing

7811 Montrose Road
Potomac, MD 20854
Monthly $69.00/year

Julian Whitaker, MD, is an advocate of a healthy, nontoxic approach to living a healthy life. The newsletter does not offer medical services, but Dr. Whitaker draws upon his 25 years of experience in the medical field to offer his opinions and recommendations to the reader. The newsletter emphasizes nutrition, vitamins, minerals, and supplements.

Dr. Robert D. Willix, Jr.'s Health for Life

824 East Baltimore Street
Baltimore, MD 21298
Monthly $74.00/year

Editor Robert Willix, MD, covers a wide range of health topics in each issue offering specific step-by-step recommendations. Mainly emphasizes nutrition. Journal sources are provided for each article or topic covered.

Melpomene Journal
Melpomene Institute
1010 University Avenue
St. Paul, MN 55104

The Melpomene Institute assists girls and women of all ages to link physical activity and health through research, publication and education. The journal is sent to members of the institute. Regular membership is $32 per year.

Midlife Women's Network
5129 Logan Avenue South
Minneapolis, MN 55419-1019

National Women's Health Network
1325 G Street NW
Washington, DC 20005

Both are advocacy organizations focusing on women's health care issues and a clearinghouse of women's health information. Individual membership of $25 per year includes bimonthly newsletter and access to a women's health information service.

Nutrition Action Health Letter
1875 Connecticut Avenue NW, Suite 300
Washington, DC 20009
10 issues/year $24.00/year

Published by the Center for Science in the Public Interest, this newsletter discusses both recommended and not recommended foods by brand name, exposes labeling deceptions, and encourages readers to consume foods rich in vitamins, minerals and other health-promoting nutrients.

University of California at Berkeley Newsletter
P.O. Box 420148
Palm Coast, FL 32142
Monthly $24.00/year

Published monthly by Health Letter Associates in
New York, this newsletter covers a wide variety of health subjects including men's and women's health issues, nutrition and
fitness. The publication also provides a Buying Guide (i.e., over-
the-counter pain relief medicines) and answers questions sub-
mitted by readers.

WomenWise
38 South Main Street
Concord, NH 03301
4 times/year $10.00/year

This quarterly newsletter presents information on
feminist topics such as the status of current legislation as well as
various health and wellness topics. The publication is supported
by the Concord Feminist Health Center.

About the Author

Susan M. Lark, M.D., is a noted authority in women's health care and preventive medicine and is Director of *The LifeCycles Center*. She also maintains a private practice in Los Altos, California. Dr. Lark has been on the clinical faculty of Stanford University Medical School, Department of Family and Preventive Medicine. She is an associate member of the Department of Family Medicine, El Camino Hospital in Mountain View, California. Dr. Lark lectures widely on women's health-care issues and is the author of two best-selling guides for women: *The PMS Self-Help Book* (Celestial Arts) and *The Menopause Self-Help Book* (Celestial Arts).

Women seeking appointments for patient care or information about lectures and speaking engagements can reach Dr. Lark through *The LifeCycles Center*. She is also available for phone consultation with women living outside the San Francisco Bay Area who would like more personalized information. Contact Dr. Lark at the Center, (415) 964-7268, for available time and fee schedule.

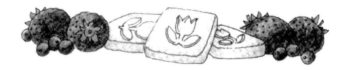

Acknowledgment

The author and publisher wish to extend a special acknowledgment to Shelly Reeves Smith and Cracom Corporation for permission to reproduce the creative line drawings found in the food section of this book. These and additional drawings, together with a collection of wonderful recipes, may be found in the cookbook *Just a Matter of Thyme* available in your local gift or book store. Inquires may be addressed to Among Friends, P.O. Box 1476, Camdenton, MO 65020 or call toll free 1-800-377-3566.

Index

breast tenderness, 126
cramps and pain. *See* Cramps;
  Pain
depression, 76, 177–78, 196–97,
  214–16, 249
diet and, 76
dizziness and fainting, 124, 127
endometriosis and, 18, 21, 25,
  26–27
fatigue. *See* Fatigue
fibroids and, 9, 11–12, 13, 85
headaches, 130, 163, 202
heavy flow. *See* Bleeding
irregularity, 217–18
lower back pain. *See* Lower
  back pain
mood swings. *See* Emotions
nausea, 202, 214
normal, 18–20, 27
ovulation, 19–20, 25, 26, 27, 87,
  178
stress and, 152
weight gain, 132, 207–11
See also Estrogen; Progesterone
Menstruation, defined, 18–19
Menus, 97–99
Meridians, 201–02
Midol, 222–23
Milk, nondairy, 85, 90–91, 94, 97,
  101, 247. *See also* Dairy products
Millet, 76, 78, 97, 102
Minerals
  amount to take, 135, 136
  by mail order, 247
  depleters of, 87, 88, 89
  food sources of, 127–28,
    140–43
  importance of, 243
  nutrition of, 127–28
  See also specific minerals
Mittelschmerz, 25
Monthly calendar, 35–59

Mood swings. *See* Depression;
  Emotions
Motrin, 223–24
Muffins, 97, 98, 106
Muscle tension. *See* Relaxation;
  Stress
Music, 162–63, 249
Myomas. *See* Fibroids
Myomectomy, 233, 234–35

Nafarelin, 228–29
Naprosyn, 223–24
Narcotics, 224
Nausea, 27, 202, 214
Night sweats, 89, 125, 126
Nuprin, 222
Nutrition
  allergies to foods, 76, 77, 85,
    131, 247
  dietary principles, 75–94
  evaluating eating habits, 61–64
  foods that help, 62–64, 76–84,
    246–47
  foods that stress, 61–62, 75,
    84–89
  gradually changing your,
    242–43
  mail-order food source, 246–47
  menus, 97–99
  recipes, 100–20, 248
  substituting healthy ingredi-
    ents, 89–94
  supplements, 121–36, 243,
    247–48
  See also Fatty acids; Herbs;
    Minerals; Vitamins
Nuts, 20, 81–82, 119, 120, 127, 131.
  See also Almonds

Oats, 76, 77, 78, 97, 104
Obesity, 9, 24, 86
Oils, 64, 82, 83–84, 86, 126, 131,
  132. *See also* Borage oil; Flax oil